TRAIN **HARD**
TRAIN **SMART**
HAVE **FUN**

Discover Your Inner Champion

TRAIN **HARD**
TRAIN **SMART**
HAVE **FUN**

Discover Your Inner Champion

BUTCH NIEVES

MR. AMERICA & MR. USA

Niche Pressworks

Published by Niche Pressworks
NichePressworks.com

ISBN-13: 978-1-946533-16-6

Dedication

To my superhero, my mom, who I have been blessed to have in my life! You have taught me how to make obstacles into opportunities … and above all, to embrace life and all its greatness and to be kind. This book is dedicated to you. I love you!

Acknowledgements

This book is the accumulation of the last 35 years of my life. Over the years, I've been lucky enough to work with some of the best people I could have possibly imagined. These special people have helped me build my knowledge so that I am able to share with you, and so many others:

First and foremost, my family. I love you higher than the sky and deeper than the deepest sea!

My mother, who taught me the meaning of true love. She has always been my biggest fan and literally made me unstoppable.

My father, who taught me to love, to work and put family above everything else.

Then, there is my beautiful sister who has always been by my side, helping me, guiding me, loving me, and always getting me in trouble with my parents when I strayed too far from my path. ;-)

My wife and my son, my reasons for living! You are both my heroes and help give me the super powers to do what I do. I could never imagine my life without you.

I would also like to express my deep appreciation and love for Donna Torres, whose love, friendship, and mentorship have inspired me and helped me, so much, for so many years.

Robert Gruskin, my bodybuilding coach, my mentor, my friend. I could never have accomplished so many championships without you!

And finally, I want to thank Bedros Keuilian, for helping me reach financial freedom and showing me how spectacular our fitness business really is!

Table of Contents

NO PAIN NO GAIN NO BRAIN

BUTCH NIEVES

MR. AMERICA'S PERSONAL TRAINING

PREFACE

I Am Not a Beast

In today's fitness world, everyone wants to be a Beast or a Spartan and feels the need to try to train like some sort of monster.

But the reality is we are not monsters. We are not Spartans fighting to protect our village from being burned to the ground, or keeping our families from being killed.

Most of us are just fighting to feel better, be more confident, and simply enjoy life to the fullest. You need a plan, you need effort and you need consistent action—consistent, intelligent action. Running into some gym and doing everything you can, all at once, without any real solid advice or plan will not do you any good.

People often say to me, "You must train like a Beast!"

And I say, "I am a father, I am a husband, I am a son and a brother and I was raised to be a gentleman. I use my intelligence and my work ethic to attract the things and circumstances I want in my life."

It's how my parents taught me to live my life—as a gentleman. So, why would I not train as such?

I believe the person who trains and works the smartest, is the person who will succeed in all things. Work and train hard, yes! But do it intelligently and with purpose. Have a plan. A good mentor or coach can help you!

The old saying, *No Pain No Gain* ends with *No Brain.*

Work and train with purpose and intelligence, and you will always succeed!

Just a cool quote I heard and it stayed with me

"He who makes a beast of himself gets rid of the pain of being a man."

- Dr. Samuel L. Johnson

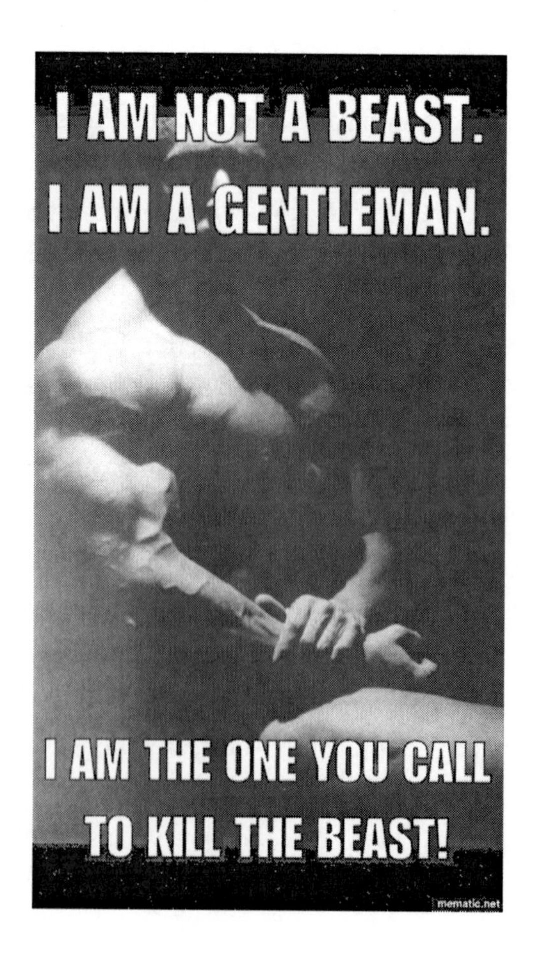

My Story:

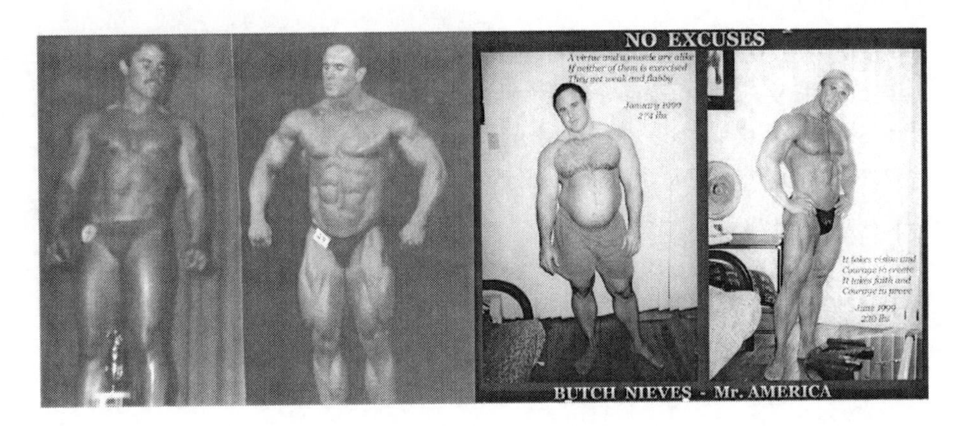

I do not have a rags-to-riches story or a sob story to tell you. I was not born with a silver spoon in my mouth but I did, however, grow up with a spoon in my mouth. This does not mean that my story does not have challenges and struggles.

I was born into a loving and caring family. My father always made sure we had food on the table, a roof over our heads, and clothes on our backs, with love and attention to spare. My mother was the matriarch of our whole family and made a warm and beautiful home for us, and for our friends to visit. When I would invite a friend over I would always say to them, "You are going to love it at my house!"

But as I said, my childhood was not without its challenges. At two years old, I was diagnosed with bronchial asthma. In the 1960s, we did not have the medications to treat asthma that we have today. So, for years, the slightest physical exertion could bring on a life-threatening asthma attack, and there were several instances when it did just that. It even caused me to start school late but, with the loving support of my family, I am here today.

The doctors told my parents that I would probably never amount to much because of my physical limitations, that they would cause me to become an introvert. I guess they never really took the time to get to know my mother!

She would have none of that! She set out to find the right doctors and nutritionist. It took years but she never quit and she never doubted that she would succeed in finding them. Four years later, with weekly injections, never missing an appointment, we finally had my asthma under control.

My mom always said if you treat people well and have faith, just ask for help when you need it, it will come! Now don't get me wrong, she did not just pray every day. She made calls every day; went to see different doctors every day; and asked other families about their challenges, every single day. And yes, she prayed over me as I was struggling to breathe, asking God to give her my asthma. Yes, she loved me that much.

Faith without action is useless. That was my first big lesson. Take action every day, have the right people around you and have faith. Believe in yourself and in the process. I became a strong, vibrant young man because of my mother's faith and because of her actions.

Fast forward to high school. I was buying my clothes in the husky department and girls were starting to look interesting to me. So, I knew I had to drop some weight. I decided to join the track team after a failed attempt on the football team, which I will discuss later in the book. Of course, being somewhat overweight I was put on the shot-put team and I did quite well actually.

But this is where I found out what I was really good at, weight training! I also noticed that the more muscles I had, the more the girls liked me and the more the other guys respected me, so I was hooked.

Now, unfortunately, in my high school we did not have the best coaches, and basically just did bench presses and a few chin-ups. Then in the summer of 1979, I joined a gym called the Muscle Clinic with my cousin and met Sam Sanchez, my first real coach. (Kind of!) Sam was the top bodybuilder around, so I watched everything he did and sought out his advice. Just like my mom had taught me, I asked for help.

He took me under his wing and gave me general advice from time to time. Then in 1982, I entered my first bodybuilding contest and won first place. I had come down from a chubby 185 pounds to a weight of 152 pounds. Truth be told, there was not much competition that day. So, was this good luck or bad luck? Hard to tell at that point because afterward I thought I knew it all, and so did everyone else around me.

You see, I basically starved myself. All I ate was granola bars and tuna fish out of the can. It's embarrassing to admit this now, but I was so naïve and had no idea about nutrition at the time. What made matters worse was that I was considered the local expert because of this contest. I started giving out free advice and telling people what to do. Don't get me wrong, my heart was in the right place, I just had no real knowledge or experience to help so many different types of people.

I kept training, I kept learning, I kept competing, and I kept training others as well. Then in 1991, I competed in a contest where I was favored to win. It was a good distance from my home, so many of my friends and family drove quite a few hours to see me win again. But this time there was real competition and real judges.

I am not sure how many of you reading this have seen a Body Building competition, but at the end of each division the emcee calls out the top five finalists for their trophies. So, I began my preparation to collect my 1st place trophy. Fifth place is called. I know it's not me, so I smile. Fourth place, I chuckle this time. Third place, I have a bit of concern but I am confident, after all, I am who I am. Second place is called and it's not me so now I have a huge smile on my face because I won again, or so I thought! Another name is called for first place I did not even make the top five. I walked away with my head hung low in total embarrassment and in complete shock!

I had been winning a lot of shows that year and felt confident that I would win easily because after all, I am who I am! (Yea right!)

That was my first mistake, being over confident! We need to be confident, yes, but always stay humble and work hard. Always be honest with yourself. The truth will set you free!

Most of the time everybody would tell me how great I was and that I was a beast and nobody could beat me. Second mistake—I listened to people who had no real knowledge and just wanted to make me feel good! I knew deep down that I was not training as hard as I should have been. I needed to hear the hard truth that I was simply not good enough. Not yet!

My third, and biggest mistake was that I did not focus on my goal. I started to do things that would affect my workouts, my diet, and recuperation. And not for the better.

It was, by far one of the worst feelings I have ever had in a bodybuilding competition.

You see, nobody beat me that day but me. Yes, I was crushed and ready to give up. But I knew that I would regret not giving it one more chance.

Thankfully, by the grace of God, I had another shot. We don't always get another chance. Always make the most of your opportunities because you never know when you might not get a second chance.

So, I made a promise to myself that I would give all I had to be my very best! If I lost, I could live with that. I was going to do everything in my power to win. I was going to eat right, train right, and have absolutely no regrets. I was going to hold nothing back. I was going to get a great coach! I was going to learn! I was going to do everything in my power to be the best version of myself that I could possibly be. And, if I was going to lose a competition, that would be fine because I would be at my physical best, and that is not a losing proposition!

I can proudly say that from 1992 to 1999 I was never again beaten in my division in the good old USA. I went to Europe several times and represented America proudly in the World Championships and the Mr. Universe competition. I always placed in the top four of over 180 national champions from all different countries! I have also won many power lifting events including the East Coast Power Lifting Championship.

Now, did I learn some new radical training method? Not really. What I learned was to FOCUS on one thing to achieve greatness. Hyper focus if you will!

The second thing I learned was that I may not get a second chance, so I approached every contest, every business venture as if it was my last. We only have so many tomorrows. Do it today! Right now, with all your heart!!!

The third thing I learned was that somebody must win; why shouldn't it be you? And don't let anybody tell you that you can't do something, especially if they have not done it themselves.

If you give your heart to something. you should fully expect to become successful.

Getting in shape is not magical, it is a simple set of rules that will turn into habits that you will follow to reach your goal and stay fit for your lifetime.

Beware of the B.S.

I want to share ONE important thing to avoid when you are thinking about starting a fitness routine.

After thirty-five years in the fitness field, I am still asked the same questions over and over. Which diet works the best? Which workout is the best? And how fast can I lose the weight?! One person says this and the other person says that. Everybody is an expert these days.

And that, my friends, is what you need to learn to avoid first, the so-called "fitness experts."

Please listen to me! Having a million Instagram followers does not make you a fitness professional. Being a celebrity does not make you a fitness expert. Fitting into a size three and having implants does not make you a fitness expert!

And truthfully, being a fitness expert does not necessarily make a person the right expert for you!

I am not everybody's cup of tea. I'd rather be someone's shot of tequila anyway! LOL

I'm kidding, I heard that joke and it made me laugh. But seriously …

I do a very specific thing. I am a fat loss expert and I do it through boot camp combined with weight training! If you want to lose weight using dance, I am not your guy! If you want to improve your baseball swing, I am definitely not your guy!

What I am trying to say here is that when you go out to find a trainer or coach or even a mentor, that person should have gone through at least some of what you've gone through in life. Or, they should have successfully helped many people with the same goals.

Here are a few things that I think you should ask yourself that will help ensure success in this fitness journey of yours:

- What are my specific goals? (We will dive into this more in the next chapter.)
- What do I want to accomplish?
- How much weight do I want to lose or gain?
- What do I want to look like?
- How do I want to feel?
- How do I want to perform?
- What is my time frame?

The answers you get will determine what diet plan you will go on and what training regimen will be best for you.

I had a great coach when I won Mr. America, Mr. USA, and the NABBA National Championships! I could have never done it without him!

His name was Bob Gruskin and he was the National Amateur Bodybuilders Association (NABBA) USA President. Legendary John Grimek, then editor of *Muscular Development* said this about him:

> In 1975, as a University instructor in Biology, teaching courses in human anatomy and physiology, and exercise physiology, Bob was amazed that the textbooks available at that time did not contain photos of well-conditioned athletes showing detailed human muscular anatomy. Desiring to complement his lectures with such material, he attended his first bodybuilding competition to obtain close-up photos of the human torso.

As time passed, Bob received assignments from various bodybuilding publications to cover competitions and do profiles on various athletes. He became a regular contributor as well as a contributing editor for many magazines, including *Muscle Training Illustrated*, *Muscular Development*, *Muscle Mag International*, and numerous foreign publications. Bob also held both an AAU and NPC national judge's card and judged over one hundred events.

During this time, Bob helped coach eight AAU Mr. Americas, five NABBA Mr. Universes, numerous AAU Mr. USAs, AAU Junior Mr. Americas, AAU Teen Americas, and professionals of many federations in dieting and posing.

The following are some of the champions Bob has coached:

- Mike Antorino – Mr. Universe & Mr. America
- Cathy Butler-Corish – Miss Universe

- Joe DeAngelis – Mr. America, Mr. USA, Mr. Universe
- Mike Duffy – American Bodybuilding Champion
- Matt DuFresne – Teenage Mr. America, Mr. USA, Mr. America
- Jeff King – Teenage Mr. America, Teenage Mr. USA, Mr. America, Mr. Universe
- Casey Kucharyk – Mr. Poland, Mr. North America
- Billy Leahy – Masters Mr. USA American Champion
- Hiram "Butch" Nieves – Mr. USA, Mr. America, Mr. USA American Champion
- Gerry Scalesse – Pan Am Games Champion, Mr. World, Mr. Universe
- John DeFendis – Mr. USA & IFBB Professional
- Victor Terra – Three-time Mr. Universe

This is just a short list of people Bob worked with.

For those who are looking for a trainer, and I think you should, ask yourself these questions.

- Who are some of their current and past clients?
- What is their point of reference?
- What are their training mythologies and strategies?
- Will they be using bodybuilding techniques, kicking boxing type workouts, or running in the park?
- Do you fit into this group?

Make sure that you are ok with it so that you can enjoy the process.

Your trainer should have studied all aspects of fitness, they should have been mentored by another well-experienced trainer, and have gone through the process themselves.

The main point of this is to take massive intelligent action with the right people to ensure ultimate success and not waste time, or worse, injure yourself! Build your super team, your army of allies!

My **Job**
Is To Get Thru
Your **Mind** and
Into Your **Heart**!

BUTCH NIEVES

MR. AMERICA'S PERSONAL TRAINING

CHAPTER 1

The Possibilities

I want to kick things off by sharing stories from some of our clients … as told in their own words. Sometimes, it's easier to believe what's possible by learning what others have already achieved.

Gissania Roman

Don't let anybody tell you that you can't do it.
Especially if they haven't done it themselves!!!!

My name is Gissania Roman, I am forty-one years old, a second-grade teacher, and mom of two boys. Time after time I started the "fitness/healthy lifestyle" journey. I tried time and time again to go to the gym and watched countless fitness videos with no success towards my goals. I gave up time and time again because of the lack of motivation, mediocre results, fear of exercises, or training that I was not familiar with. Never had I achieved anything close to what I received when I walked into New York Fit Body Boot Camp three years ago.

The second I walked in, I was greeted by this burly man who emanated power and confidence. Initially, it was a very intimidating feeling attending his boot camp session. Day after day, I stood in the back, hiding in the corner to avoid eye contact, feeling like that hid me. Little did I realize each time I went, even though I feared the spotlight, I was stepping into one. Each time I went to boot camp I felt stronger and stronger not only physically but mentally I was overcoming all my limits.

He has a way of scaring you and making you feel so strong and powerful at the same time. The results rapidly increased and my motivation was at a high I had never anticipated. I decided my goal of simply losing weight wasn't enough. I decided to train one-on-one with him.

I got great nutritional advice, educated training advice, and someone who actually cared about helping me achieve my goals the smart way. What I mean by the "smart" way is that every training session consisted of teaching me each body part, how it needed to be worked, using proper form, and always trying to avoid injury now and in the future. The one part of training I did not even take into consideration, but he gave me, was the motivation. I've come to realize I am my own worst critic.

When training, nothing was ever good enough for me, I strived only for perfection. I voiced this constantly with Butch and he constantly

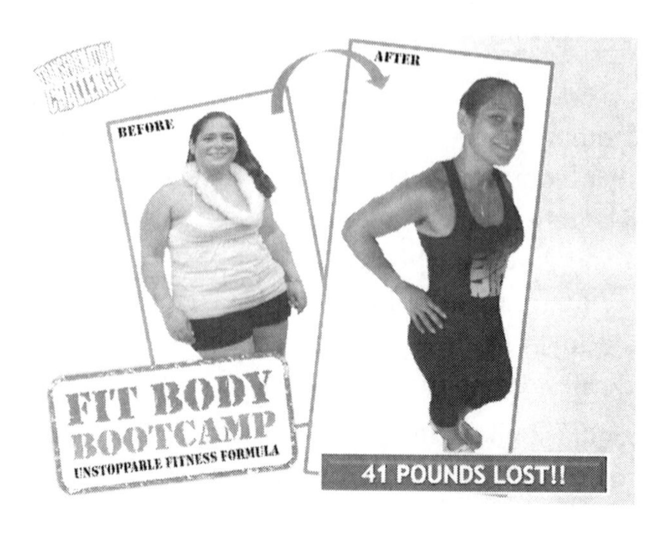

reminded me to enjoy the process and focus on my goals step by step. He also reminded me that goals are always changing depending on my progress. Plain and simple—no one is perfect!!!

One day during training, he asked me, "What is your favorite body part?" It was a question I will never forget because it translates to everything I do. In my impossible quest for perfection, I said, "My arms or maybe my shoulders." I also went on to say what I was unhappy with until he stopped me to ask, "Do you want to know what I think your best body part is?" Of course, I was waiting to see what he thought so I could start working on it immediately and he simply said, "Your heart." Two simple words made such an impact on me. He explained, "You have the heart to work hard, stay dedicated, accept both triumphs and challenges, and continue to strive every day for more. If you don't have heart, you will never achieve anything. Celebrate your strengths!"

Any time I question myself, or the process with my fitness journey, or things that happen in life, I think of this conversation and push through.

You walk in one day to lose some weight and three years later you continue to get stronger and stronger, physically and mentally. I've accomplished so much in these three years besides just losing weight. I try my best to live a healthy lifestyle for myself and for my family. I share my love for eating right, training hard, and crushing goals with my family. We all do it together.

I could not have done that without the help and knowledge of Butch Nieves. He has openly shared his expertise with me from the first day I walked in, afraid, to today, when I feel like I could conquer the world. I continue to be grateful.

Marc & Marilena Viscogliosi

The beginning of our journey with fitness and Butch Nieves was first traveled alone—by myself. There was some apprehension from my usually supportive husband, Marc, about my new endeavor. In all honesty, it was understandable, seeing that every attempt at losing weight was never a permanent one. I had reached the pinnacle of my own frustration, and his uncertainty in my newest undertaking added fuel to my fire. I tend to enjoy "proving them wrong," so off I went to do just that.

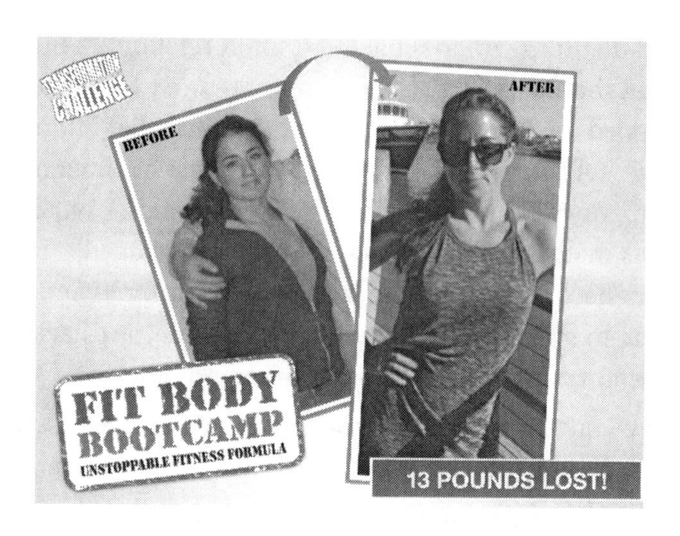

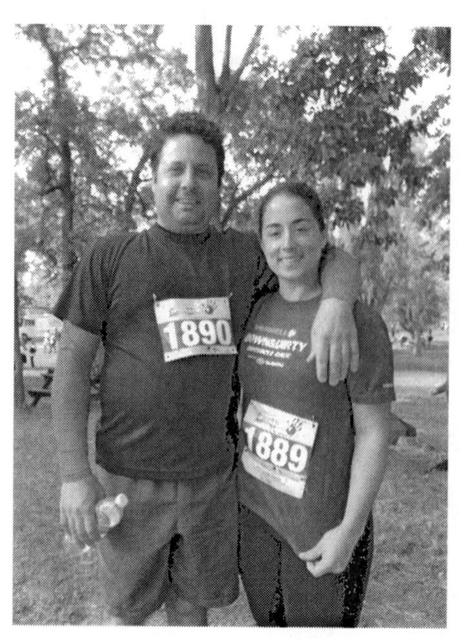

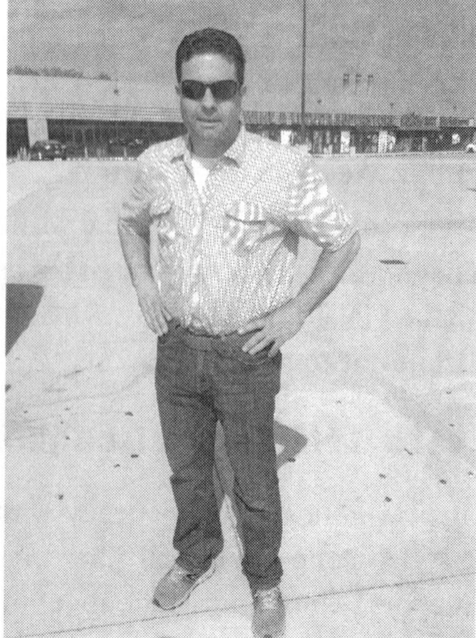

This time it stuck. It was a journey of patience and faith. Before dawn, my feet would hit the floor and I headed over to the gym. Back row on the mat—I watched, I learned, and I listened. The changes happened and everyone noticed which was even more motivating.

More friends followed and joined, more incredible transformations happened. Knowing how spirited, strong, and adept my husband Marc can be, I patiently waited. I was aware that when his heart was ready, it would be his turn to achieve amazing results with Butch Nieves. So, it was eight months later Marc decided to join me and learn what it REALLY took to change your body. His results have been unbelievable. Marc is now more adept, confident, and thriving not only physically, but also mentally.

For Marc and myself, it's been wonderful. I LOVE that we now share this passion together and are on a path to better health as one. Our "date nights" sometimes consist of hitting the gym and encouraging each other to new limits physically. Our conversations are peppered with statements like, "Wow, I can't believe I actually managed to do that!" or complimenting and the other with "Babe, you killed it in there today. I'm so impressed!" When our sessions with Butch Nieves are over, we leave happy, lively, and strong, but most importantly, feeling even closer to each other.

Ariel Lewis-Ballester

I was overweight, unhappy, depressed, did not feel attractive, and had just gotten out of a six-year relationship. I decided to take some action and change the things that I did not like about myself and I chose to start with my health.

From my education, I knew how to eat healthy and clean, but clearly, at 215 pounds, I was not very good at applying it to my life. In part, because I was comfortable and convinced myself that, the pressures and requirements from graduate school made it impossible for me to cook and eat healthy—excuses.

Yes, I told myself I was making excuses and I was the only architect of my mental and physical well-being. I stopped pointing fingers and owned up to my own deteriorating health. I knew that going to the gym to exercise was not the right approach for me since I had tried this in the past and failed because I did not know what I was doing. I know metabolism, I know food, and I know math. Without asking for help and without even knowing the term "meal prep," I stopped drinking alcohol, quit added sugars, and started cooking healthier versions of the foods I enjoyed eating.

I divided my daily calories into five balanced meals, each meal had a vegetable, a protein, and some type of carbohydrate. It wasn't always easy, but in three months I was able to lose 35 pounds while not doing any form of exercise aside from my daily walk to and from work.

At this time, I knew that I had to incorporate exercise into my life if I was going to keep improving and if I was going to be able to keep the weight off. I knew nothing of exercising other than my failed attempts, which meant that I needed to seek help.

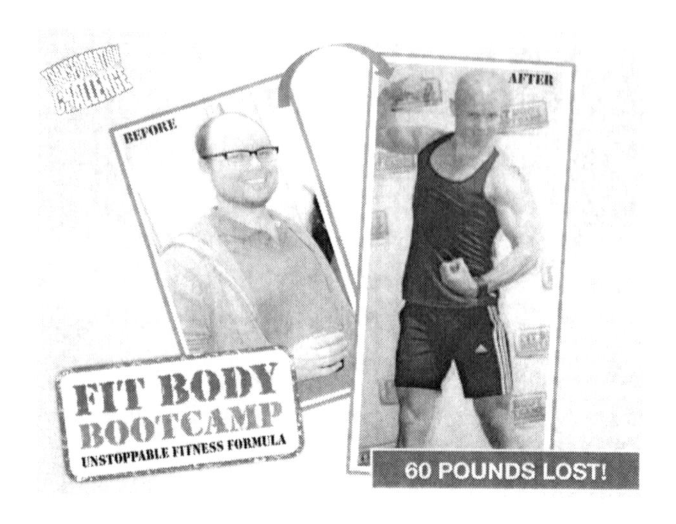

I bought a one-month subscription to New York Fit Body Boot Camp and I signed up for the beginner class. I was nervous and excited when I first walked in through the doors, but soon I was just excited since I saw the group was mostly composed of women. I told myself I'm probably younger than they are and I don't seem to be in worse shape than they are. This will be easy.

The instructor, which turns out is Butch Nieves, yells, "LINE IT UP AND START JOGGING IN PLACE." I saw him cracking jokes earlier, he's probably a nice guy, this for some reason validates my initial assessment. JUMPING JACKS—so far so good! AIR SQUATS—this can't be any easier! HANDS OFF PUSH-UPS—oh, crap. What is this? I can't even do one push up! The realization of how wrong I was starts to set in. JUMP SQUATS—a squat and a jump. I got this! Nope, I don't got this. Legs start to burn almost immediately. I can barely jump an inch off the mat and from here on out struggle after struggle.

I lack strength, I lack stamina, I lack endurance; what have I gotten myself into? I constantly stare at the door thinking of excuses after excuse to run away. The woman standing next to me looks at me, our eyes meet and she says, "Come on! I do one, then you do one." She's clearly in pain, but she's not stopping. That gave me the push to finish the thirty-minute session, even if I was constantly failing.

I did feel some feeling of accomplishment in that I stayed until the end, but I felt defeated and beaten. I did not finish the workout. How could I allow myself to reach this state that I am in? I wanted to be able to prove that I could do everything that that trainer was yelling. I wanted to be able to say, is that all you've got? So, I kept coming for more and in a month, I lost another ten pounds.

I was getting better, but I still lacked strength, stamina, and endurance. I wanted to get better, be more fit, be able to do push-ups on my toes. With the help of Derek, one of Butch's trainers, I incorporated weight training into my routine and almost immediately, I noticed the increase in my strength. I was addicted to feeling great and seeing the changes in my body and in my mind. I gained back my confidence, I didn't feel depressed, and I was finally happy; which goes to show that body and mind are connected; working on your body improves your mental health and vice versa.

My journey taught me many things about myself, but I think the most important lesson I have learned was something Butch told me, "You have to surround yourself with people that motivate you, people that expect the very best from you, and people that you admire and strive to be like." Unknowingly, I had done that when I recognized that I needed help with my fitness.

I decided to be that person for others. I approached some of my family and friends and made myself available to them to help them achieve their health goals. With the help of my friend, role model, and mentor Butch, I became a fitness instructor and trainer. This has given me a larger platform to impact people and pay it forward with my knowledge, motivation, and friendship.

I educate myself almost on a daily basis by reading about nutrition, diets, fitness modalities, and exercises. I also a pay close attention to other trainers to learn from them. I participate in different types of classes. I use the tools that I learn to help others achieve their goals, be it nutrition-, health-, or fitness-related. I never get tired of seeing someone else be able to achieve their goals because that means a healthier individual that will also influence someone else and help them become a healthier version of who they are.

Maria Castro

I started at New York Fit Body Boot Camp because I was overweight and out of shape. I came in and immediately was greeted with smiles and welcomes. There were people of all sizes and fitness levels, which made me feel comfortable. As class began, other members around me were correcting my form and giving me tips along the way.

As a few of us started together and were on the same path we began pushing each other to do better on the mat. The trainers would ask me what my goals were and give me guidance on my fitness routine and meals to help me achieve those goals.

As my fitness progressed and the pounds dropped, I met more and more members. Each one had a similar story, just at a different point of their journey. The more I wanted it, the more people around me rallied for me to get there. I realized that these people were my boot camp family. It was only right that I too paid it forward to new members as they came in.

In five months, I was able to drop 37 pounds. I was so proud of myself. I had not only achieved my goal, but I had also found a support system along the way. Life went on and slowly I started going back to my old ways and missing boot camp. Eventually, I had gained almost all the weight back. Upset with myself I said, "Enough is enough" and headed back to my boot camp. With my head down and in shame, I walked back through those doors. To my surprise, I was once again greeted with smiles and welcome backs. No judgments, no shaming, all support.

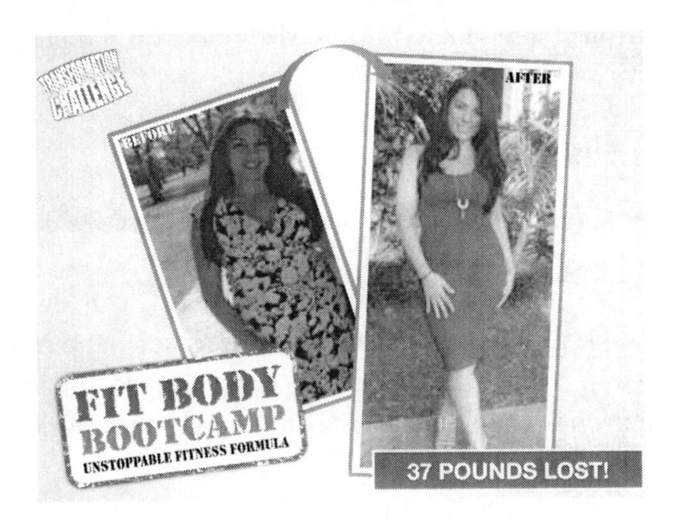

I fought my way back to my prior fitness level. I lost the weight again. I have come back stronger than before. But the most priceless part of all, is that my boot camp family was there to cheer me on along the way again. Bonds became stronger. Support grew bigger. Now I know I am unstoppable. Now I know this is a lifestyle, not a temporary weight loss. Now I know the true value I have in my FBBC. I challenge anyone to find that at their gym! Thank you for everything you have done for me, on and off the mat.

Jackie Rodriguez

The results speak for themselves! Butch has created an environment conducive to success, and I am a better and more fit woman because of it. He has decades worth of fitness knowledge and experience and it's one of many things that sets him above the rest.

Jennifer Ferro

It's been about four years since I have started my journey at this amazing place. I can't say enough about the trainers, the team, and the environment. I have made lifelong friendships with this second family! Don't be intimated by it. Take the first step and walk through the doors of this amazing place and talk to the knowledgeable team there. I promise you won't regret it!!!

Erica Rodriguez

I have been training with Butch and his team since 2013. I honestly cannot say enough good things about my experience with them. They have not only made me a stronger and healthier person, but they have helped to change my whole mindset. I have become a happier and better person inside and out because of their expertise and support. At Mr. America's Personal Training we are a community that works hard and supports each other.

John Marano

Butch is the real deal. It does not matter if you are a novice, he will show you the way to look and feel like a million $$$.

Dan DeNapoli

Mr. America isn't a part time trainer, he's all in. He will transform anyone who has the will to commit themselves to him. Butch will motivate you towards changing your life forever. This man has literally a half century of experience and he's constantly evolving, a truly deserving Everyday Champion. Commit to Mr. America and enjoy your new journey.

Tracey Beets

I first met Butch when I became a member of his original Butch's Gym, which was located in the Bronx back in the 90's. In today's time where health clubs, gyms, personal training studios, and personal trainers come and go, Butch somehow manages to always hold the line and keep driving forward. Butch has years of experience in the fitness industry, his knowledge alone is priceless. If you're serious about getting into shape or just losing a few extra pounds, then it would be highly recommended that you stop in and speak with Butch. Trust me when I say you will save a fortune, and most importantly, if anyone can help you achieve your fitness goals it would be Butch. Best of luck.

If you'd like to read more inspiring success stories
from our clients, you'll find them on our website at
MrAmericasPersonalTraining.com.

What's Necessary:

EFFORT DISCIPLINE HEART

BUTCH NIEVES

MR. AMERICA'S PERSONAL TRAINING

CHAPTER 2

The Promise

"We all must suffer one of two pains: the pain of discipline or the pain of regret! The difference is discipline weighs ounces, while regret weighs tons!"

-Jim Rohn

I will be giving you a GPS, if you will, for your fitness journey. As long as you stay on track, I can guarantee you will reach the body you want. But it will take effort, discipline, and heart!

You will also need the right group of people around you, your dream team or an army of allies. These people will have the same mind-set as you do and will want to improve their lives and yours.

You will also have the naysayers and you will have the enablers. The naysayers are the people that will say you can't do it or you are not good enough or that it's just too plain hard. They may say that they know a better way. Blah, blah, blah. Just like the quote from the previous chapter, **don't let anybody tell you that you can't do something, especially if they haven't done it themselves!**

To me, the enablers are the most dangerous. They mean well and might even be close family members. Their mantra is, "You don't have to work so hard," or "You can take a day off." Or my favorite, "that's good enough!" That my friend, is loser's language.

The enablers will say, "Hey, it's your birthday," or "It's my birthday," or "It's a special occasion." Any excuse to take a day off and not work towards your goal or not work at all. It seems all too common these days, that for many people the goal is to not work hard or, to not work at all. We'll talk more about enablers again later, for now remember that just because they live a life full of excuses doesn't mean you should.

My father loved his job and loved to put in a good, hard day's work. He always told me that it made him feel great and that I should love to work hard, it's a blessing and an honor.

Here is a story from my childhood that really showed me what my father taught me about character:

When I was around eight years old, my father had come home from a full day's work and the whole family; my mom, my father, my sister, and I were sitting down for dinner, as we did most nights. My mom casually asked my father how his day went at work. He then told my mother that he had gotten a new job and would be starting the beginning of the following week.

My mother, a bit surprised, said to him, "Wow, that's quite sudden." Without hesitation, my father said, "Not really, I lost my job two weeks ago!" Then an eerie silence fell over the dinner table. You see, my father had left the house every day at the same time, and had come home every day at the very same time for the past two weeks, as he had when he was working.

My mother then said to him, "Angelo Nieves, where have you been going then?" She said to my father, "You have called me every day at lunchtime to say hello, check on the kids, and to let me know when you were coming home, and you were not at work?!"

My sister and I looked with our eyes wide open at my father because when my mother used your full name it meant she was not happy and you were in big trouble!

My father reached into his pocket and took out a new business card with all the new information of his new job. You see, back in those days, my father was an independent consultant and computer programmer. That meant he would be hired to set up a certain system and then when he was done he would have to look for a new job.

What my father said next to my mother I would never forget!

My father told my mother, "I did not want you or the kids to worry, so for the last two weeks **my job was to look for a new job**. I spent eight hours a day doing just that. I took lunch at the same time and came home at the same time until I found a job!"

"I love my family," he said, "so I make sure to support them and protect them every day!!"

Being a bodybuilding champion, many people asked me who my idol was growing up. Most people would assume it was Arnold Schwarzenegger or Steve Reeves but I always said I have only one idol, my father!! This story was just a little taste of why. My idol, my dad, who taught me so many things. The value he placed on enjoying hard work is such an important aspect of a fitness lifestyle.

You must have a strong work ethic if you are to have any chance of success.

Stay focused on your goal to win the body and life of your dreams.

Here is a challenge and a few simple strategies that will point you in the right direction. They follow the **KISS** principle, if you will, **K**eep **I**t **S**imple **S**illy!! ;-)

First, My Challenge to You

Give yourself three months to turn your body, mind, and spirit into the superhero of your life.

Make yourself a priority, don't let anybody distract you from your goal. There are no more holidays, no more vacations, no more days off, and no more excuses!

Now, the strategies that will get you there:

Set Yourself Up for Success

Plan Smart ~ Average people plan the wedding more than they plan the marriage. Don't be average! Prepare everything and take massive action!

Set Goals ~ Write them down and be as specific as you can be! Also, put a time line on them. Goals provide focus. You will be surprised what you can do when you focus! Make sure the goals you have will make something of you to achieve them so it's ok to think big. The confidence you will develop will make you unstoppable. (We will go into further detail in another chapter.)

Get Support ~ Family and friends will be the biggest and most important part of your army of allies! Surround yourself with an uncompromising group that only gives and demands the best! A 2011 study published in *Psychology of Sport and Exercise* found that the exercise habits of people you know have a positive influence on your own exercise habits.

Here's a funny story that highlights the type of allies you don't want:

> There are three men stranded in a small rowboat in the middle of the ocean. Suddenly, a genie pops up and grants them three wishes. Each man has one wish so they must choose wisely. The first man chooses to be on a tropical island with plenty of food, money, and to be surrounded

by beautiful women. Poof! He is gone from the boat. The second man wishes to live in the big city and be a billionaire. Poof! He is gone. The genie then asks the last man what he wants. He says, "I feel lonely and want my friends back." Poof!! The two men are back in the boat!

If you don't already have a good network of people who will be your fitness allies, join us at Mr. America's Personal Training and New York Fit Body Boot Camp where we're happy to give you the support you need to achieve your goals.

Invest in Yourself ~ Never be cheap on yourself—you are worth it!

Make the Commitment ~ Just simply decide that you will do this and nothing will get in your way! You will find solutions to all obstacles.

Forget the Past ~ Don't let your past influence your future. You have learned from your past mistakes, and you now know what you no longer want. Write down the things you will no longer do and don't allow anything to stand in your way. Then, alongside each item, write down what you are now going to do in its place. This will help to reduce the influence of past behaviors and increase the chances that you will be successful in reaching your goal. Share them with your allies and go forth confidently and as **the superhero of your own life!!**

Never Say ~ "I can't, we'll see, I never will, if only, or it's good enough." This is losers' language as we said before and negative energy. No room for it in our lives!

Believe in Yourself ~ If you ask an adult if they can jump over a car, they will say no. But ask a child and they will say, "I don't know, I haven't tried yet." Let's bring our inner child back and believe again!

Here is a poem that my mother gave me before I went into high school, she said she did not know who wrote it. But I believe in my heart she wrote it for me.

It might be a bit corny for some of you but I find it to be 100% true!

You never know
Until you try,
And you never try
Unless you really try.
You give it your best shot
You do the best you can.

And if you've done everything
In your power and still fail
The truth of the matter is
That you haven't failed at all.

When you reach for your dreams
No matter what they may be,
You grow from the reaching,
You learn from the trying,
You win from the doing.

The main point is this: **When your goal is believable to you, it will happen.** If you don't really believe your goal can be achieved, but you're hoping it might, it never will.

The road to Someday leads to the Town of Nowhere!

Believe in your dreams and let's DO IT NOW!!!!

PROGRESS
NOT PERFECTION

BUTCH NIEVES

MR. AMERICA'S PERSONAL TRAINING

CHAPTER 3

What are YOUR Goals?

As discussed in the previous chapter, it is very important to have very explicit and time sensitive goals.

So, the first thing to understand is clarity. You must be crystal clear on what your goal is! Is it to lose twenty pounds, to run a half marathon, or to be able to ride a bicycle with your grandchildren? When you know what it is, write it down and put it in a place you will see every morning when you rise, and every evening before you go to sleep.

Second, putting a time frame on your goal gives you a sense of urgency. Activity does not always necessarily mean progress. So, make sure you have a few short-term goals to chart your progress. Also, it's great to have a special date attached to it like a birthday or a wedding, or maybe a planned vacation—sort of your bodybuilding contest date! Not that you are going to get on a stage or prance around half-naked but hey, you never know! LOL

This is why I like the twelve-week time frame, if you need that much. Some people only need four or six weeks to reach a great fitness level; it all depends on where they are starting. This is why a great coach can help assess your physical condition and help you set up a good time frame to reach any fitness level.

One of my fitness goals was to be considered in good shape by my peers, even when I considered myself out of shape.

Third, you must know why you want to reach that goal, the benefits of reaching your goal. This will keep you going when the going gets tough, and help you focus on the prize.

Fourth, you have to figure out what is standing between you and your goals. If you did not have some kind of barrier, you would have already attained your fitness goals. Is it procrastination? Is it crazy work hours? Or is it simply being lazy? Whatever it is, figure it out!

The fifth one has to be finding the people or organizations you need to work with to get there. In this way, they can help you set a specific plan of action to help you attain your goal! They are also very important part of your army of allies and as such, will be as critical to your success as your friends and family.

What enabled me to be successful as a competitive bodybuilder and an entrepreneur was my ability to ask the best experts I could find for help! My army of allies was very important, and it still is!

Now the sixth one can throw a wrench in the whole thing simply because your goals may change as you change. **Understand that as your fitness level increases, your confidence will too!**

As your knowledge of fitness, nutrition, and what your body and mind is now capable of grows, your first goal may seem, well not enough! So be somewhat flexible, as long as it makes you better!

Always challenge yourself and take a risk, anything worth something will never be easy. Just a word of caution, your goal should not be shallow, it should mean something to you deeply to attain it or you will never maintain it!

Les Brown, a great motivational speaker, has said the problem with most people is that they engage in low-level thinking and low-level goals. And even worse he says, they hit those low-level goals and think they are getting somewhere. He goes on to say that you must be willing to risk or you cannot grow. And if you cannot grow, you cannot become your best. And if you cannot become your best, you cannot be happy and if you cannot be happy what else is there?!

When I started training, my goal was never to become Mr. America or Mr. USA. My goals were simply to get leaner and receive more attention from the girls.

As I developed physically and mentally, my goals changed and I believe your goals will too. I am not saying you will want to become a bodybuilding champion. In fact, I would advise you against it. The competition aspect of bodybuilding is just not healthy.

My present goal is to help as many people transform their lives as I can. I no longer train competitive bodybuilders because I feel it's more important and a better use of my time to help someone transform their life than to chase plastic trophies.

I do believe in my heart that as your confidence grows in leaps and bounds, it will affect all aspects of your life in such a positive way.

The confidence I attained from being in great shape, and the discipline I learned, helped me start my own business and live an amazing life.

Now, the last part of designing your goals is accepting responsibility. What I mean by that is, they are YOUR goals! They are not anyone else's goals. They are your responsibility and you cannot expect everyone around you to understand why you are doing what you are doing. Do not get upset when someone does not understand or help. Simply keep moving forward and away from those people.

Always remember your goals are your vision of your own future, and the better you feel the better you will live!

At the end of the day, you are the one that has to want it!

LIFE IS NOT A MATH TEST!! IT'S ABOUT **HEART!**

BUTCH NIEVES

MR. AMERICA'S PERSONAL TRAINING

CHAPTER 4

What is Your Why?

huffpost.com

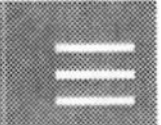

HUFFPOST

> “
> **Your heart will get you through the tough times and through the negativity and disappointments that you may encounter from time to time.**
>
> —Butch Nieves of New York Fit Body Boot Camp

What's pulling you, the real reason?

Most people come into my studio and tell me the doctor told them they need to lose weight, or that they simply don't feel well and want to get back into shape. Sounds good, right? Wrong!

Everyone has that X Factor or special reason that they want to lose weight and feel better. I have never forgotten a story a client once told me after close to a year of training him. He originally told me that he had wanted to get a little stronger. I was like sure, no problem.

We started training and he trained hard, ate well, and never missed a workout session. He was very dedicated and it showed! He dropped a considerable amount of weight and his strength improved by at least

30%! A win-win, so I asked him one day, “What drove you to be so dedicated and consistent?”

He finally gave up the real reason. He was an accountant working at a client’s home office. This client had a small closet safe where he would walk in and store important papers and such. When my client went to put the paperwork back into the safe, he had to push himself through the doorway, and this is where he got stuck. He tried everything but could not get himself out. The fire department had to be called and they had to break down the walls to get him out. He said it was the most humiliating day of his life! He swore right then and there it would never happen again!

Your X Factor must pull you towards your goals, not push. It will be the reason you can get up so early, because you have such a compelling reason to do so! We all hear people that say, “I am not a morning person,” but it’s because they have no reason to get up. They live in survival mode and are okay with that.

This book, my studio, and my team do not live in the survival mode that the average and basic people live in. We, my friend are not average, it’s not why you purchased this book!

It is my job to get through your mind and into your heart! You see, I believe that life is not a math test, it’s not based on numbers and facts. We all have limitations thrown at us, but it’s the person with the most heart that will eventually reach their goals.

I truly believe that we are amazing creatures and the only disability is a broken spirit!! You have that divine choice to decide what happens next because you are not broken!

I often ask my clients what is their best body part? They ponder it for a while and say, “Oh, I like my legs or my arms.” I ALWAYS tell them, “NO! It’s your heart, because without heart you have nothing and you will not be able to get through the challenging times in your life.”

It takes a tremendous amount of heart to go against the norm and fight for your dreams! There will be times when you just want to give up and quit. There will be times when common sense tells you to give up. There will be times when you simply just want to stay in bed and do nothing but you won't because you want this and you are not average, you are not basic. And the reason why is simply because you and your family are worth having a powerful YOU!

One of the most asked questions I get is, what is better or more important for losing body fat, weight training or cardio? My first reaction is to say boot camp because I own one, and we have gotten amazing results for thousands of our clients. But the technical answer is both. Weight training first, then cardio. (We do both in our boot camps.)

But here is the real truth, whatever you enjoy doing most will yield you the best results. So, let's say boot camp is not your thing and spin is, by all means do that, because if you enjoy it and you put your heart and soul into it, you will yield better results. If Zumba excites you to go more often, then do that. You see sometimes, it's not what you do, but how you do it that matters!

No matter what or how you choose to get yourself back in great physical condition, you should learn to love it and the things it affords you to do. In that way, it never really feels like a chore and it's something that will pull you to do it!

Several years ago, I had very successful and amazing client. He owned a rather large construction company. When he first came to me he was overweight, stressed out, and always tired. I put together a cross training routine for him to do that yielded him amazing results, but he also did his part by eating well and keeping active when he was outside of the gym.

In no time at all, he lost thirty pounds, gained strength, and had tons of energy! He believed in the training so much that he made it mandatory for several of his managers. Most of the managers did so well, they got great results and they loved it. But there was one manager who just hated being in the gym, and guess what, he did not get good results.

Now you might think that he did not train hard, well he did train because I made sure of it. Unlike my client, he did not do his homework and he did not have the right mindset or attitude. His goal was to get it over with and get on with his day, period! He had no fitness goals and just felt like the training interrupted his day instead of improving it.

Like I have said throughout this book, you have to want it for yourself and you have to be ready to do it. You must know in your mind that this is the smart thing to do and know in your heart that this will improve the quality of your life and the lives of everyone around you!

Train Hard and Win Easy, My Friend!

EXERCISE BUILDS.
DIET SHARPENS.

BUTCH NIEVES
MR. AMERICA'S PERSONAL TRAINING

CHAPTER 5

Limitations?

"Fight for your limitations and they will be yours forever!"

- Brian Tracy

First, let me teach you how to get fat! Wait a minute, what did you say? We all know that most everybody wants to lose weight, but that's not what their habits say.

Here are my top five fat-gaining tips:

1. **Skip Breakfast!**

   This will slow down your metabolism and make you one cranky ass person. Since you need at least 50 grams of carbohydrates for your brain to just be able to function, it kind of makes you … well, not so sharp either!

2. **Do Not Drink Water!**

   Since water helps in breaking down fat and keeps the system flushed, it also helps you recuperate from training sessions. Why would you want to do that if you are looking to get fat?

3. **Drink alcohol on a regular basis!**

   This is a super great way to get fat. Your body needs fuel to burn during workouts, and if alcohol is in your system, the body will burn that first and not the fat you are carrying. Just saying!

4. **Eat Infrequently!**

   Again, this will slow down your metabolism and lead to binge eating. A sure way to get fat!

5. **Do not work out hard, or use any training system at all!**

   The HIIT System (High Intensity Interval Training) is one of the best systems to burn tons of calories and speed up your metabolism and promote one healthy and outrageous body! So, don't do it if you are looking to get fat!

Well there you have it, the best tips I know on how to stay or get fat!

If your goal is to get into your best shape and you are doing any of these things my advice would be to stop immediately! I mean if you really want to get out of the average zone!

Hold yourself to a higher standard.

Most people around you will tell you to not be so hard on yourself, and that it's okay to take a day off and eat all you want. It might be, but first let's earn that choice and second, make sure you are living the life you want to live, not the life somebody else thinks you should have to make them feel more comfortable.

There are a Few Very Important Things I Need to Ask You ...

Are you in?

There will be obstacles, there will be haters, and there will be days that you just want to give up. But those are the days you must remember why you started in the first place and remember how far you have come.

Are you in? Cause I am! This is what this book is all about! I am totally invested in helping you reach your fitness goal!

Do you believe?

You must trust in the process and trust in your hard work. I believe if you follow the simple strategies outlined in this book you will be successful. But you must believe in yourself. I believe you can and will do it!

Are you committed?

Are you going to do all that is required of you? Train hard, eat well, and sleep enough? Plan and prepare? And do it consistently?!

No More Excuses!

---

ex·cuse

an attempt to lessen the blame attaching to (a fault or offense); seek to defend or justify.

We might as well talk about our excuses because we all have them. The problem with excuses is that they never bring you closer to your goals and they are only designed to make YOU feel better!

Excuses do not make anybody else feel better. And no matter how valid they are they never get the job done!

Try this exercise: write down your top ten excuses. Here are the ones I hear all the time:

- I have no time.
- I have no money.
- I am too old.
- I am too tired.

- I don't feel well.
- My joints hurt.
- It's too cold out.
- It's too hot out.
- I have too many things going on in my life.
- I have no help from anybody.

> "Instead of saying "I don't have time" try saying "it's not a priority," and see how that feels. Often, that's a perfectly adequate explanation. I have time to iron my sheets, I just don't want to. But other things are harder. Try it: "I'm not going to edit your résumé, sweetie, because it's not a priority." "I don't go to the doctor because my health is not a priority."
> If these phrases don't sit well, that's the point. Changing our language reminds us that time is a choice. If we don't like how we're spending an hour, we can choose differently."
>
> -Wall Street Journal

Successful and confident people know that regardless of how many excuses they give, it will not help them or anyone else achieve any worthwhile results.

Even justified excuses will not help you reach your goal. When things go wrong, and they will, the successful person will see it as an opportunity to learn and fix the problem. While another person will use it as weapon to quit or give up and spend most of their time and energy on whining and making even more excuses!

Good old Les Brown said, "If you want to keep getting what you are getting, then keep doing what you're doing!"

Let's make a pact here and now. NEVER use the excuses you have just written down and always look for a **solution** instead of an excuse!

The Peanut Gallery

Okay, so we all have relative and friends that try to enable bad eating habits when we go out by saying things like:

- Go ahead and have that piece of cake.
- Come on, just one drink. (But it never stops there.)
- What's wrong with you? You have changed for the worse.
- You can have one slice of pizza, can't you?
- There is no need to go to the gym, you can take a day off.
- You look great already, enjoy a little.
- You have become so boring.
- What do you mean you are not having a drink at my wedding?

What do you do? How many times can you tell someone no? Do you lie and say, "Hey, I am a recovering alcoholic and can't drink?" Do you say you're a diabetic and really can't eat that cake?

Hell yes! Do whatever it takes to stay on track. Some people just will not listen to reason.

First and foremost, always eat before you go to an event. This will cut down on your appetite and any chance of messing up your diet.

Second, you can always call ahead and ask if the food can be specially prepared for you.

Bring your own food? Sure, why not? I mean how bad do you want it?!

One of my clients' biggest struggle has been how some people say to them, "Wow you have lost a lot of weight, you're getting too skinny." The negative/positive comments.

I always say, "Remember where those comments come from, the peanut gallery!" Their opinion of you is none of your business.

The next three months is your very own life-changing transformation; do not let anybody or anything get in your way. Always remember one thing: successful people don't focus on how hard the work is, but rather on how great the results are!

A Few Simple Healthy Strategies to Keep You From Making Excuses:

- Go to bed early and wake up powerful.
- Go to sleep and wake up consistently at the same times every day.
- Eat five to six small, healthy meals every day.
- Eat breakfast every day.
- Minimize simple sugars.
- Drink 48 to 64 ounces of water per day.
- Do at least three cardiovascular workouts and three strength workouts per week.
- Learn to say **NO!** Don't put yourself in a place where it takes you away from your dreams!

Make Exercise Automatic

Step 1: Make Exercise a Priority

Step 2: Make the Time

Step 3: Assign the Time

Step 4: Do It!

Remember to reward the behavior, not the outcome. Reward yourself for working out or walking five times this week, NOT for losing a pound. Celebrate your victories no matter how small they may be, they are all important!

Don't sweat the "skips". Inevitably, real world obstacles will occasionally come between you and training. Don't sweat it. Once you've committed to exercising daily for the next seventy-five years, missing a day here or there isn't catastrophic. View the skip as a rest day or just that—a temporary skip and go on from there. You can get back on track quite easily.

In today's world, we have so many distractions with social media, cell phones, iPads, and even that annoying voice on your shoulder saying to let it slide yet another week. This is when your army of allies and your discipline need to kick in full force because all those distractions can only stop you temporarily, only YOU can stop you permanently!

Want more great health and fitness tips like these? I put several on a special bonus page just for our book fans. You'll find helpful videos, meal plans, fat-melting diets, training routines, and more at **http://MrAmericasPersonalTraining.com/Resources**

Number One Rule:

EVERYTHING MATTERS!!

BUTCH NIEVES

MR. AMERICA'S PERSONAL TRAINING

CHAPTER 6

Focus

Let's focus on three rules:

Rule #1—Everything Matters!

Everything you do, or do not do, matters! Every workout missed matters, every little cheat snack or missed meal matters. Your fitness relationship will be the most brutally honest one you will ever have. If you are not doing something right, your body will let you know! It's that simple!

If you are not hydrating enough, you will feel weak. If your nutrition is off, you will have no energy and have trouble sleeping, and you will not be able to recover for your next workout!

Take time to plan and prepare your nutrition, you cannot out-train bad nutrition. Every choice, every thought, every action, matters!

5 Action Steps to Staying on a Healthy Meal Plan

1. **Weigh yourself every morning.** Preferably at the same time and on your own scale. Now let's keep in mind this is not the only measure, it does not tell you if you are a good husband,

wife, or parent, BUT it does tell you if your weight is going in a direction you may not want to be going. Studies have shown that people who weigh themselves often are more likely to control their weight.

2. **Write it down.** Keeping a log of your food is the best thing you can do to control your weight and eating habits. There is no guess work, it's in black and white.
3. **Plan it out.** We have all heard the saying *if you do not plan, then you plan to fail.* This is extremely true for planning your meals. Ask yourself, "Do I know what I am going to eat? When am I going to eat? And how much? Even, "Which restaurant is a better choice?"
4. **Prepare.** Make sure your home is stocked with the proper foods, so you eat on time and don't binge on the wrong stuff. Spend a day and prepare your foods if you are cooking your own meals. I take a Sunday and grill a bunch of chicken and prepare other foods and then arrange them in plastic containers. A few are frozen and ready for the week.
5. **Have the right tools for the job.** If you are traveling with your food, have a good food carrier to keep it warm or cold. Have a quality scale to weigh your food and calorie counting book to be able to know how many calories you are taking in.

Rule #2—Take Consistent Action

Very often a person will walk through the doors of our studio and say something like, "I just saw your place and have been thinking about getting back into shape. I was wondering what you have to offer." After we go through a short presentation and show them all the benefits of working out and doing it with us, a few people will always respond with "Let me think about it!"

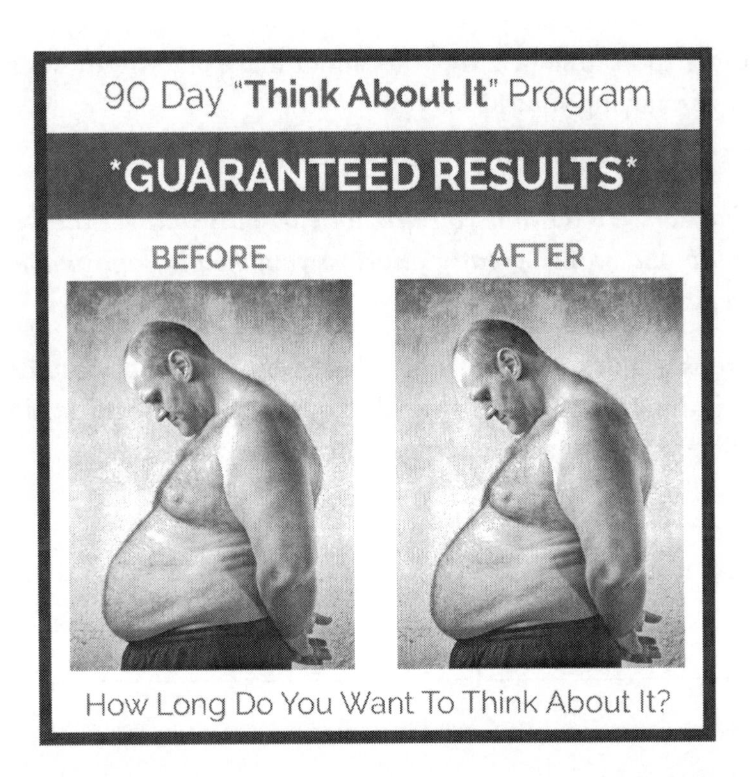

Then I will reply with, "How long have you been thinking about it already?" They usually smile and say a very long time. I then say, "During that time, have you gotten into better shape?" Of course, they say no. I tell them that they are no closer to getting in shape than they are right now—**let's do it!**

If you do not take action, even the biggest intentions will do absolutely nothing! You must take some sort of action. At first, it can be a small thing, like taking a walk, maybe working out twice a week, or eating healthy breakfast, and slowly things will start to change. But, if you take no action, nothing will change for the better!

We must make that distinction. The longer you do not take care of your health, the more damage you can be doing to your body. Think of your body as a bank account; if you do not make any deposits in the way of training and eating healthy, you cannot make any withdrawals down the line of enjoying your life as you get older.

This is a great question from Brian Tracy:

What can you do that you are not currently doing, that would be easy to do and would greatly improve your health, and maybe even your wealth?

Here is a quick game changer. Take your time and write down at least five things that will answer that question and begin to do them immediately. This simple action can change everything.

1 ____

2 ____

3 ____

4 ____

5 ____

Let's break Rule #2 into 3 parts:

Part A: Take Consistent, Intelligent, Massive Action

The things that no one in the fitness industry wants you to know or talk about, including trainers or gym owners, is what you really need to succeed with your fitness journey. And the reason they don't want to talk about them is that they can't sell them to you. There is no profit in it.

There is no magic pill, no magic diet, or super special training routine. Why? You see they all work! That's right, they all work. Whatever you stick to will work to some extent.

So, the first thing no one can sell you is your own consistent action.

No matter what type of workout you do, if you do it long enough, you will see some kind of results.

If you make it consistent, intelligent action the results will be even better.

Learn and study about the results you want. Learn from a proven mentor or great coach. I did and became Mr. America and a successful businessman.

But, let's go one step better—if you take **consistent, intelligent, and massive action**, your results will be better and faster! You will be able to enjoy an amazing life with your family and friends. Do all you can with all your heart and soul!

So many people say to me, "I wish I started this sooner." And, I always say, "As long as you started and never quit, that is what's important and that's what matters."

Part B: Give it Consistent Effort

The second thing no can sell you is effort. Effort truly is between you and you! Only you know if you are giving your best and doing all you can. And this is why it's great to be around other people like yourself who want the same things you do and demand more than just average results.

I always train with the best people that I can find so I can become my best. You must be comfortable with being unconformable!

Part C: Live by Consistent Discipline

The third thing you will need is discipline. It is easy to go the gym when you feel good; it's easy to do things you need to do when you are feeling great and have lots of energy. That's what the average person does, they wait for the right circumstances before they begin anything. But the moment they break a toenail or have a bad hair day, it's no more gym and no more goals!

This is where your discipline comes in. This is when you need to remember why you started!

Rule #3: Have Patience with Yourself and Trust the Process!

As we have discussed before, you should celebrate every victory no matter how small. They are all important to your long-term goal! Now don't get me wrong, I am not saying going out and eat junk or drink yourself under the table. Celebrate with a new dress or great experience doing something you could never do before. Do things that enrich your life and others; it will be so magical for you and those around you.

You will also go through injuries. We all get them from time to time. But do not lose heart, depending on what your injuries are, your job will be to heal and nothing else. Don't let ignorance out-think your common sense. Go to a reputable doctor that understands what you are working towards and follow his instructions to the letter so that you can get back to training at the intensity you need to reach your goals.

Now, by all means I am not saying to stop all training because your shoulder hurts. Get your shoulder checked out by a doctor. Until you are healed, we can still train other parts of your body and get in plenty of cardio. Where there is a will there is a way. Just be smart about it!

TO CHOOSE
THE ACT IS
TO CHOOSE THE
CONSEQUENCES
OF THE ACT

BUTCH NIEVES
MR. AMERICA'S PERSONAL TRAINING

CHAPTER 7

My Concern

Fearless Fitness or Foolish Fitness?

I remember when I was a young bull in the gym tearing things up, there was always an older guy telling me to be careful, to avoid injury, and to take care of my joints. But if I didn't, time would have a way of slowing me down.

Well, now I am the older guy in the gym telling the younger guys to slow down and take care of their joints. The old saying is really true, *Youth is wasted on the young.*

This is why I strongly suggest to get a great coach and listen to what they have to say. Learn and use their advice so you do not do damage to your body and you do not waste the most precious thing you have—your time! You will never get your time back. Always ask yourself, is this the best use of your time? Trust me, every time I ask myself that, it makes my day so much more productive.

Today, I also see alarming new trends towards fitness. With the hugely financially successful Spartan and Tuff Mudder Mud Runs, and CrossFit Centers popping up all over...there are an enormous amount of under-qualified trainers entering the market and with them, an increasing injury and fatality rate!

Wait what did I say? Fatality? Yes, people are actually dying in the name of fitness! When any fitness program has death attached to it, it just might be a good idea to stay away from such an activity. Just saying.

There is something wrong when you take certain aspects of fitness and turn it into a dangerous force.

Certain exercises are meant to improve the body's performance in athletic competition and/or functionality. But when you make the exercises themselves a competition, it can and often is completely dangerous.

I have seen so many people run these races and then need weeks and weeks of recovery where they can do little to no physical activity at all. They are just too beat up from the race. I have also personally seen some very serious injuries; one injury required amputation, and the other several complex surgeries so the person could walk again. Does this sound like fitness to you?

And oh yeah, if you finish you get a medal, no matter what, everybody wins right? Wrong! I totally get that this might be in someone's bucket list or from coach potato to Spartan kind of thing, but let's think bigger than that, let's have goals that make us better, not just beat us up!

Your goal should improve your life and the lives of the most important people around you. Work toward something like that and you will feel a sense of pride you have never felt before, I guarantee it!

I have had the great fortune to work with an amazing coach recently. What she told me summed up what any kind of coach must always do. She said I must inspire you, that I must encourage you to keep going, but I also must equip you with the necessary tools to make you reach your goal!

I want to say thank you to Nicole for all you have done for me. I feel like a better person having gone through this process with you!

My goal was to inspire you and encourage you in the book and as a gift, in a later chapter I will equip you with all the tools you need to reach your fitness goal!

Does that sound like a good deal? Sure it does, because you would have never gotten this far if you were not in it to win it, so to speak.

Here are three rules that I have always used in my personal life and in business that have served me well. Not sure where I got them from but I never forgot them:

#1 Always do what you say.

#2 Always finish what you start.

#3 Always stay humble and say thank you!

This is your journey, your time, and your body. You only get one body so treat it right. I will say this—if you want to train for hours and hours, I am not for you; If you want to risk your health and wellbeing, I am not for you; If all you want to do is work out all day, three times a day, I am not for you; If you want twice the results in half the time, like my friend Josh Carter says, "Then I am your guy!"

Also, after training thirty-five years, I believe there are three important factors of a great training program:

1. **Variety**—Keeps you from hitting plateaus, and most of all, boredom.
2. **Intensity**—Know your intensity levels to avoid injuries while still making progress. The old saying, "No Pain, No Gain," ends with "No Brain." Train hard, but train smart. Recovery is just as important.
3. **Consistency**—The body thrives and responds to consistency. When you stop working towards the things you want, the things you don't want start to take over. Sound familiar?

Training facilities such as a Fit Body Boot Camp have all these key components in their programs.

You can find several of my favorite workout routines and tutorial videos under the Bonus Content that goes with this book. Go to
MrAmericasPersonalTraining.com/Resources
to register your book and get the bonus videos.

NO GUTS
NO GLORY

BUTCH NIEVES

MR. AMERICA'S PERSONAL TRAINING

CHAPTER 8

What's Next?

The time was August of 1982 and I was sitting in a big box gym with a few of my powerlifting buddies. One of them was a mountain of a man named Nat Servino. Nat weighed in close to three hundred pounds and was ranked top ten in the country in powerlifting. Like I said, be around the best and you will become one of the best.

One of his best lifts was an 805 pound squat which blew my best squat of 710 away like it was nothing. My nick name for him was Pound Cake; you see we would eat an entire pound cake before our heavy days of training so we would have plenty of carbs in our system. Hey, I told you I was not so bright at the beginning of my career! Nat called me Fruitcake because he would always say I was crazy for doing bodybuilding competitions because we could not eat cake!

But back to my story, we were sitting in the cafeteria area they had at the time, and I was telling them about an opportunity to buy a small, badly equipped gym. But I was nervous about it because I was afraid to fail.

You see, everyone at my job at the time said I was crazy because I had a great position, with great benefits and paid vacation. What's better than that, right?

This box gym that we were training in at the time also rented spots out to other small businesses. This one girl had a small hair salon inside the gym.

Try to picture this: She walks over to us twiddling her hair and chewing gum and sits down at our table as if she owned the place. Now, there were three of us sitting there when she came and interrupted our conversation. Altogether, we probably weighed over seven hundred pounds.

Without any fear in her eyes, she looked at me and said, "You looking to open a gym?" I did not even know her very well but I said, "Yes." And she said, "You would have to compete against this gym." After I told her that didn't bother me, that I could handle it, she said, "Good, then let me ask you one more question." Nat looked at me and said, "You are on your own, buddy," which I kindly thanked him for.

So, I said, "Shoot, what is it?" I thought to myself, *what could she possibly say to me that would mean anything at all or even make any sense?* She said, "Do you think you are good enough?" Without hesitation I said, "YES!" and she said, "What's your problem? Stop talking about it and go do it!"

I opened Butch's Fitness World on October 3, 1982, and it became the bodybuilding Mecca of the Bronx, yielding many champions!

So, I ask you, are YOU good enough? Don't you deserve a great life? What are you waiting for? Let's do this!

Always remember, there will be people who live in survival mode because it takes no effort. People who just want to get by day by day and never want to be criticized. Don't be one of those people! It's okay to be criticized, be comfortable with it. It's the only way you learn and grow. Remember, change is good!

I have also had people walk through my door looking to change their life and tell me, "I want to lose weight and look great but I don't want to sweat and I do not want to work hard or too intensely."

First, intensity is a relative—you determine what is intense for you at your current fitness level. If you choose to go forward with your fitness, your intensity will rise as your fitness level improves. After three months, most of our clients chuckle at their first workouts and always say, "Boy, I thought those first workouts were hard, but they are nothing compared to what I can accomplish now."

I will say this, if you are afraid of sweating or refuse to train at 70 to 80% of your intensity, your results will be limited. Can you still lose weight without intense training? Absolutely, but it will take twice as long and you will just be a thinner version of yourself, not a stronger or better version.

Earlier in the book I said I am not everyone's cup of tea and I meant it. I do not like lazy people and refuse to be around them. What I do is not for everyone. You see, I do not have a single, cookie cutter fix-it-all plan and I don't pretend to. We let everyone try our boot camp three times so they can check it out, but we are also checking you out! I want to see if you are the person we want in our fitness family. Ask yourself, are you the kind of person other motivated people want to be around? And if not, then this might be a good time to change that.

It is said that one of the quickest ways to make friends is to complain about something, everybody wants to play the victim and join in and say, "Poor me." Not anymore, not for you!

Another thing is that so many people are looking for the Magic Bullet. Everyone is looking for a quick and easy thing to buy to help them lose weight. What can they drink, what can they eat, what pill can they take to make all their fitness goals happen?

But as you know now, you already have all you need to get into the best shape of your life—your mind!

Think of it this way, remember that concert you really wanted to go to or that pair of boots you had to have or you would die? I bet you did everything you could to get them, didn't you?!

Ask yourself again, "Who and what do I need to get into better physical condition?" Then be resourceful about it.

What are you still saying? Working out is hard?!

Try diabetes, try heart disease, or try cancer! Now that is hard! Did you ever lose someone because of those diseases? I did, and there is nothing harder than that. Try losing days at a time because you are laying in the most expensive bed in the world, a hospital bed!

Most of us think it's hard because we just are plain lazy. And, more importantly, it's just not that important to you, and one day, it may be too late. The one thing that makes us different from animals is that God gave us the power of choice. I say this with much love, don't be lazy and make the right choice for you and your family!

The truth will set you free, my friends. You see, you can have anything in life you want, you just can't have everything. If you want to live on the couch, eat pizza every day, hang out all night long: you can do those things, sure. But—great health will never be yours. You deserve to have a great body, not another drink. With a little discipline and above-average thinking, you can be very successful.

Don't tell me you don't have time; I say bullshit to that! How many Facebook posts do you make a day? How many TV shows do you watch? Oh yeah, how is your favorite sports team doing? Such a waste of time that you will never get back. Remember to ask yourself, "IS THIS THE BEST USE OF MY TIME?"

To do more of one thing you must do less of another. And if that is sleep, so be it. Wake up thirty minutes earlier and skip some rope. There is so much you can do if it's really that important to you! No more excuses!

Focus and don't hold back!

My goal in this book was to give you simple strategies that you can implement right away, to see results in a reasonable amount of time, regardless of what fitness level you are!

Remember No Guts No Glory! DO IT NOW!

BUILD YOUR ARMY OF ALLIES

BUTCH NIEVES

MR. AMERICA'S PERSONAL TRAINING

CHAPTER 9

My X Factor

In Chapter Four, we talked about "Your Why" and your "X Factor." Before we discuss getting started, I want to share my X Factor story with you.

When I started high school at Mount Saint Michaels in the Bronx, I went out for football. I still remember the first day of practice. After the first play of the day, I bent over to pick up the downed football and BAM! I got spiked in the back by the captain of the football team. His name was Stanley.

I thought my back was broken, and I could not play the rest of the game or the rest of the season for that matter.

I so wanted payback on Stanley, but I had to get stronger.

When I could finally move without too much pain, the only thing I could do was lift weights. So, I ventured into the weightlifting room to try to lift weights.

The first day in my high school gym, the very first person I ever saw lifting weights was a boy named Tommy Cara. He was bench pressing. I did not know it at the time, but that is just about the only thing the kids did back then was bench press. We did not know any better and unfortunately, neither did the coaches.

Tommy you see, was pressing 405 pounds for reps as a sophomore in high school. I thought that was normal. I was wrong.

I did not know that Tommy was a monster bench presser and had won just about every bench press contest there was. What did I know? I thought this was average!

When I tried the bench press for the first time, I started with an Olympic bar, which weighs 45 pounds by itself, and two 45-pound plates which came to a total of 135 pounds. After all, Tommy had four 45-pound plates on each side so this should be easy for me. Yeah right!

My friend helped me lift the bar to try my first rep; when he let go of the bar, it almost split me in two! I was amazed at how weak I was compared to Tommy. If he could do it, so could I.

So, I started bench pressing almost every day. I had no idea about recovery and sadly enough neither did anyone else. But I was young and healthy, so I could take the pounding of training every day. It still wasn't a smart way of doing things.

I did improve quickly and reached a max press of 225 pounds by the end of my freshman year. Then I joined the track team and did shot put and javelin. This is the first time I had the chance of working directly with a coach. While he did the best he could, he did not know much about training. He did show that he cared, and he gave his best every day.

As luck would have it, that damn Stanley came back to haunt me. We could not be in the same space together; he would always try to bully me and any other freshman he could. He would throw javelins at the freshmen, thinking it was funny. If you don't know what a javelin is, it's basically a spear. He would put an empty bottle at the end of the javelin and try to throw it at us. Every time we saw each other, we would get into some kind of fight.

While he was older and bigger than me, I benched 225 pounds, and I thought I was a bad ass. I was wrong. Luckily, there was always somebody there to separate us.

I told myself that one day I would pay him back. I swore to it, no matter how long it took!

Stanley was a year ahead of me and finally graduated high school and was out of my hair. I had stopped any sort of training my senior year, which was 1979, because I had started to notice girls and cars!

So, I went to work to be able to afford both. And for the next few years, I worked on cars and became a mechanic. After a few really cold winters and working outside in the airport, I knew this was not for me.

Life is Full of Surprises...

So, let's fast-forward to 1996 when I owned my second gym called Iron Kingdom in the Bronx, to get to the point of my story.

It was a place where I made lifelong friendships. One particularly good friend was a crazy guy named Leo. He was a mixed martial arts fighter and a very tough guy. He needed to get even stronger because when he fought, there were no weight classes and barely any rules. Leo wanted to train to be able to beat up the bigger guy in the ring. Yep, I told you he was crazy and he still is!

Over time, he went from a client to a close friend. I helped him get stronger and he helped me with my standup fighting, which was great because I started training Relson Grace Jiu Jitsu in 1999.

We sparred and trained together hard for six years, and shared stories about our pasts. I even told him about my high school bully and how I would love to meet up with him now and make him pay.

As it turned out, Leo also had someone in high school that he could not stand. We often laughed about what we would each do if we ever bumped into that "one guy" today.

As life would have it, that would become a reality!

One day, Leo and I were getting ready to spar when a regular gym member walked into the gym with an **M** on his shirt. Leo looked at him and said, "What the hell is the **M** for?" The young man said, "It stands for Mount Saint Michaels High School." And Leo responded, "Hey, I went there too!"

"NO WAY", I exclaimed. *"ME TOO!"*

I was completely shocked, just stared at him and then asked him when he went there. *I knew we were about the same age so, if we went to the same high school, we had to have been there about the same time, right?* Leo told me he was there from 1974-1978, that he played football, and was even the captain of the football team! WHAT?!

He then went on to tell me that "Leo" is his nickname and his real name is Stanley! I told him, "You have to be kidding me." He said, "No, why?" I never told Leo my bully's name, and he never told me the name of the person he hated.

You see, my real name is Hiram and my nickname is Butch. We both had nicknames, we were both bald by this time, and of course, twice the size! Leo said, "You are Hiram?!"

We both looked at each other in disbelief as we discovered that we were each other's nemesis in high school! We truly hated each other for years and often spoke of how we would like to get payback.

How could this be? I trained the one person that always tried to beat me up, and I trained him to be bigger and stronger!

Leo trained his enemy to be a better fighter! Now remember, we were supposed to spar that day. My Jiu Jitsu coach was there and said, "Wow, I can't wait to see you guys go at it now!"

Well, we were both in such shock that we did not spar that day. Actually, we also did not speak to each other for several days.

When we finally did talk, Leo asked if we were still friends. "Of course," I said, "Damn you got lucky!" We both laughed while still in shock. How could we have helped the one person we couldn't stand for so long?

Leo and I always really focused on our training and asked very little questions about each other's pasts. Honestly, we just did not care about the past, we only cared about training. The training is what our friendship was based on.

I know this probably would never happen to women, they simply ask more questions than men do, and have a much better memory as well!

Leo is still one of my best friends and we laugh about this all the time. He now says that he gave me the incentive to become Mr. America and I owe him a huge dose of gratitude! He may be right but, we never sparred again!

When I really think about it, maybe Leo was right. Maybe that experience in high school was my true X Factor and is what drove me to become better! I never wanted to be bullied again and never have been! I believe we need to use everything we can. Learn from our mistakes and grow from them. Use them to make you stronger and better than you were before.

You've got to find your X Factor too; that thing that gets you up in the morning, keeps you going, and drives you to be a better person every day.

Life gives you so many chances to do the right thing and sometimes it does not matter who is right or wrong; all that matters is that you do the right thing.

It's time you do the right thing for you and for your family.

It's time for you to go forward and become the person you know you can be and make the most out of what has been given to you!

This is your time, stop wasting it with procrastination. We only have but so much time. Let's make the most of it!

I know you can do it,

I know it!

I know it in my heart!!

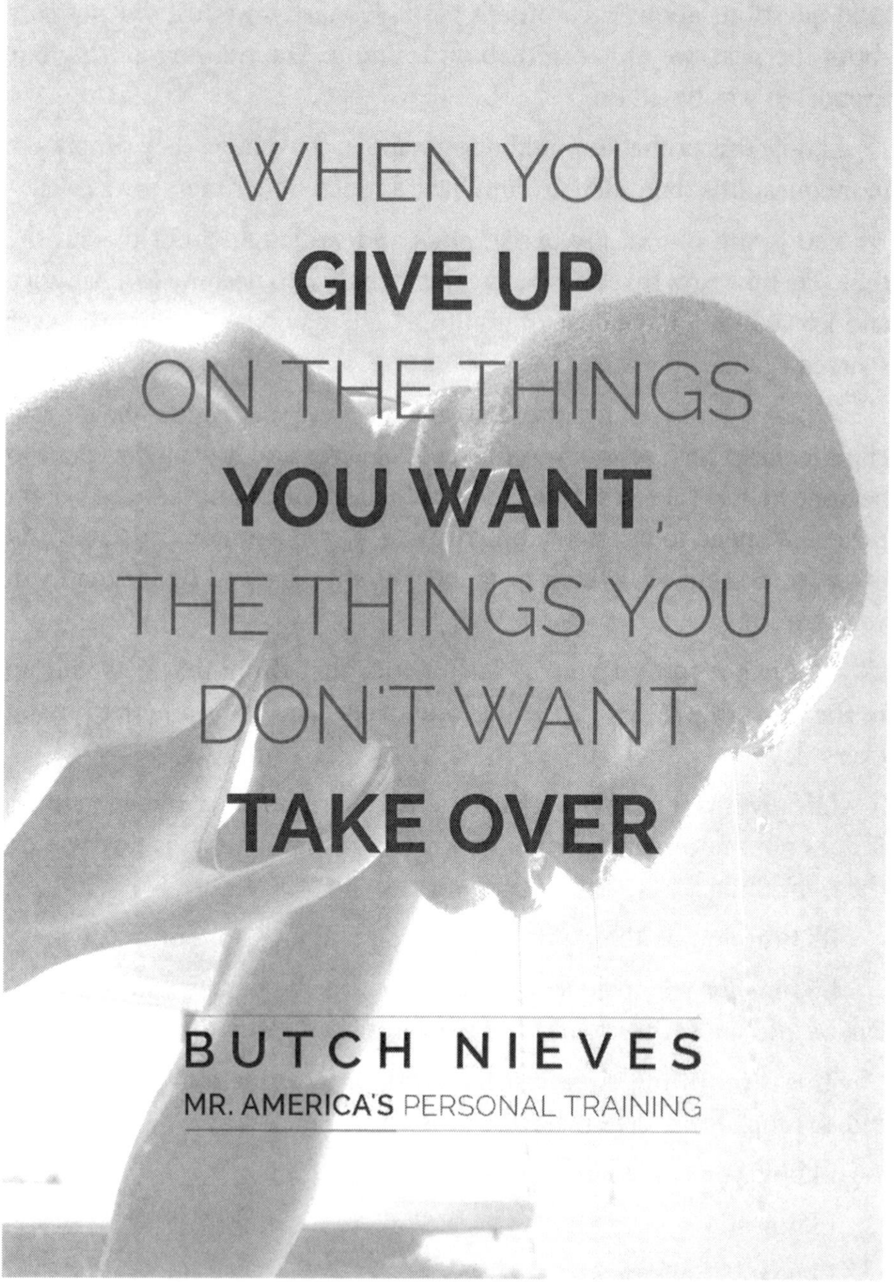

WHEN YOU
GIVE UP
ON THE THINGS
YOU WANT,
THE THINGS YOU
DON'T WANT
TAKE OVER

BUTCH NIEVES

MR. AMERICA'S PERSONAL TRAINING

CHAPTER 10

Take Massive Action

Okay, so you are ready to start your new fitness routine but it's been a while, or you are new to fitness. So, this is what we need to do.

First, have your gym bag ready the night before. (The basics)

- Loose fitting shirt and pants. Make sure they are breathable.
- Water and a light Gatorade. (You may need a little sugar lift during the workout; the light version of Gatorade is great for this.)
- A good pair of sneakers. Not an old pair, to make sure you have a good base.
- A towel to wipe all the calories away you will be burning. It's also good gym etiquette to wipe away your sweat.

Second, get a good night's rest and make sure you are hydrated. In other words, drink lots of water the day before!

Third, you should not have a large meal at least ninety minutes before your workout. You can, however, have a small yogurt or fruit about twenty to thirty minutes beforehand. Don't worry, you will burn the sugar off during the workout.

Fourth, if you are working out at a studio or local gym, I believe the workout starts when you are on your way. I like to get my mind ready and listen to some motivational music, or motivational speech before I get to the gym.

As far as the workout goes, I believe you should be training for a half hour to forty minutes, three days a week; with a combination of circuit training for the first two to three weeks.

Research has shown that thirty minutes of daily training can provide an equally effective loss of weight and body mass as sixty minutes.

Here are three simple rules to keep you training safely:

- Never work through an injury, work around it.
- Take your time; speed is your enemy when working with weights.
- Focus on your form. The movement should look comfortable.

Common Mistakes to Avoid

Mistake #1: Doing it on your own.

Instead: Find a workout buddy who will help motivate you and help keep you from missing workouts. Hire a professional fitness coach or supervised group training. A professional will assess your current fitness level and help you develop a safe exercise program depending on your goals. It's about accountability and commitment.

Mistake #2: Doing too much too soon.

Too many people think, "If a little is good, then a lot is much better." Wrong! You will risk injury and derail all of your fitness goals. Go at a steady pace and do not push yourself to failure; keep this pace for three weeks. After this time, depending on your progress, you will be ready to intensify your training.

Mistake #3: Not warming up.

Instead: Take the time to warm up properly. The main benefit to warming up is to prevent injury. Get that blood pumping to areas of the body. This lowers the chance of a muscle pull or joint injury and preps your system for peak output. Warming up also prepares the mind and body.

Top 10 Tips To Burn Fat & Achieve That Lean Look Faster

You want to fuel your body with proper nutrition with frequent small meals. Your metabolism is like a campfire. If you don't keep feeding the fire with logs, it will go out. But on the other hand, if you put too many logs on the fire you can smother it and the fire goes out as well. You have to just put the right amount in and the fire will burn strong! Feed your body what it needs and when it needs it, it will return the favor with one sexy, healthy, look and feel!

1. Use plain vinegar or lemon juice on your salads or to cook with. It helps to burn body fat.
2. Use low calorie whole wheat bread instead of white bread. Your body will utilize it better.
3. Keep in mind that people who want to lose weight should limit their bread intake.
4. Never eat butter, mayo, or other high fat spreads. Real fruit jam or mustard is acceptable.

5. Never, never add salt to your food! This will keep your water retention down.
6. Broil, bake, or steam your food. Never fry! Frying kills all the nutrients and will add empty calories. Remove the skin before cooking chicken.
7. If you have cravings for sweets, eat fresh fruits in the morning or before a workout, but never before bedtime.
8. Keep a record of what you eat. This can be an eye-opening experience. Tracking the time and quantity will let you and your trainer know exactly how many calories you are taking in. It will keep you accountable and act like a diary.
9. Eat three small meals and two snacks about two to three hours apart. A snack can be a handful of almonds or small piece of fruit.
10. Never ever miss a meal; a missed meal will set you up for bingeing.

Bonus: Drinks lots of water! Three quarters of the volume of muscle tissue is made up of water.

- Aids in the breakdown of fat.
- Keeps the system flushed.
- Helps you recuperate from training sessions.

Here is a simple way of explaining your meals and how you should eat.

Most people eat in the form of triangles. They eat a very small breakfast or nothing at all. Then they eat a medium-sized lunch. And then, the average person eats a large dinner because they are starving from not eating most of the day.

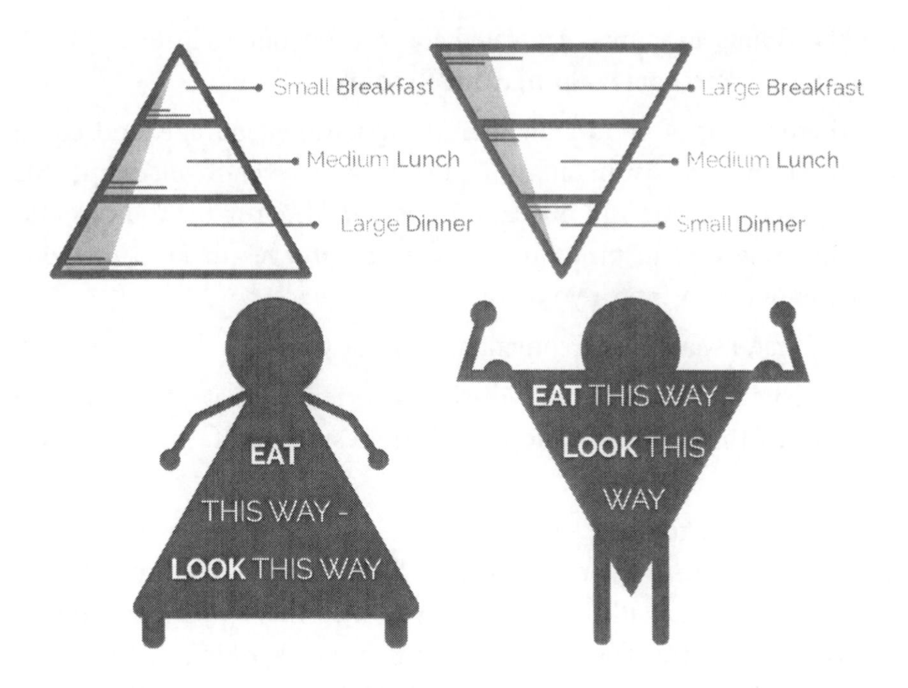

What you should do is eat a large breakfast, a medium-sized lunch and a small dinner! Also, add two small snacks every few hours.

This way, even if you don't eat the best of foods, you have all day to burn them off. The person who eats a large dinner at night has little or no chance, since most of the time the only exercise they get is using the remote control.

Get Started

So, there you go. Everything you need to get started on your fitness journey. The best way to predict your future is to create it, as we know. So, I want to thank you for taking the time to read my book by giving you several special things to help you get started. If you live near the Bronx area, check out the Skinny Jeans Special Offer on one of the last pages of this book. For all of our readers, be sure you also check out the Bonus Resources I created for you on our website at **http://MrAmericasPersonalTraining.com/Resources**

There's a lot of good stuff there to inspire, encourage, and equip you to Train Hard, Train Smart, and Have Fun...even if you're not able to work out with me and my team in person at our gym. You can also download several inspirational quotes and images to keep on your smart phone or print for your wall.

But first, I want to share my final wish for you:

I wish that you welcome all the experiences that you will have with your fitness journey and take those results and fashion yourself a great life.

I wish from my heart to yours that you pay it forward and help others, not just with their workouts or diet, but with their lives. When you help someone with their health, you help them with opportunity and confidence. This is so much bigger than just working out. I tell my trainers, help build their lives, not just their biceps. Trust me; there is no better feeling then that! A chance to help improve someone's life is such an incredible thing.

I wish for you to have a powerful resolve. Jim Rohn's definition of resolve is promising yourself that you will never give up! So never break your promise to yourself or to your loved ones.

And finally, I want to thank you for giving me the opportunity to help you become better so you can go out and make a difference and help others!

To love what you do and feel that it matters—how could anything be more fun?!

~~The End~~. **The Beginning!**

IT'S NOT **WHAT YOU DO**, BUT HOW YOU **DO IT!**

BUTCH NIEVES

MR. AMERICA'S PERSONAL TRAINING

About Butch Nieves

Hiram "Butch" Nieves was born on December 11, 1960 in New York City, NY. At the early age of two, Butch was diagnosed with asthma. For years, the slightest physical exertion could bring on a life-threatening asthma attack. With the loving support of his family and a deliberate and measured plan in place, Butch embarked upon a journey that would not only keep him healthy and strong, but would add excitement and achievement to his life. That journey was fitness and bodybuilding.

When Butch started, he was 153 pounds. At 5'8", Butch's best competition weight was 230 pounds at approximately 3% body fat.

Among the more notable bodybuilding events Butch has won are **Mr. America**, **Mr. USA** and the **American National Bodybuilding Championships.** He also placed in the top four at the **Mr. Universe** and the **World Championships**. Butch has also won many power lifting events including the **East Coast Power Lifting Championship**.

Since 1999, Butch has studied Gracie Jiu Jitsu. He has attended private classes with world renowned fighting champion Master, Relson Gracie.

Butch has been a guest on many TV shows, including Good Morning America, New York One, ESPN, Late Night with David Letterman, and Boriqua Fitness. He has been a featured guest of the Puerto Rican Day Parade, as well as many cable fitness shows and dozens of Fitness and Bodybuilding magazines.

Since 1987, Butch has owned and operated his Fitness Centers. **With thirty-five years of personal training experience**, he keeps busy with guest appearances, numerous seminars, and charity events. **Butch has earned a solid reputation for getting results, and providing patient and articulate instruction, with some clients traveling far to acquire.**

Butch Nieves can be reached at:

MrAmericasFitness5@gmail.com

Mr. America's Personal Training

3229 E Tremont Ave; Bronx, New York, NY 10461

MrAmericasPersonalTraining.com

NewYorkFitBodyBootCamp.com

And don't forget to say hello on Facebook:

Facebook.com/ButchNieves

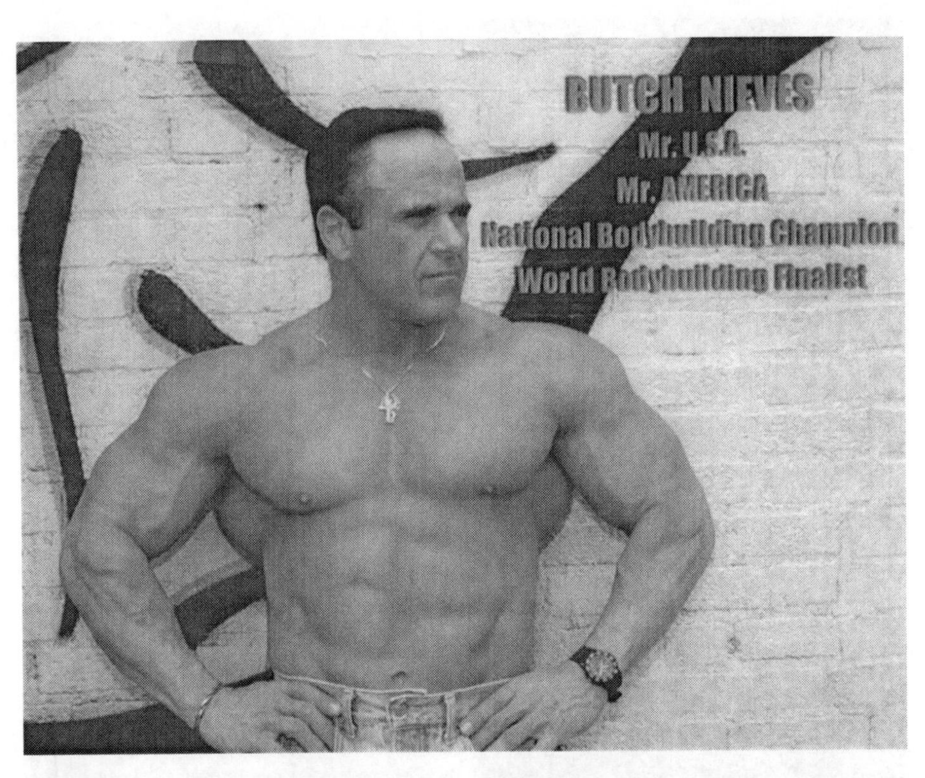
BUTCH NIEVES
Mr. U.S.A.
Mr. AMERICA
National Bodybuilding Champion
World Bodybuilding Finalist

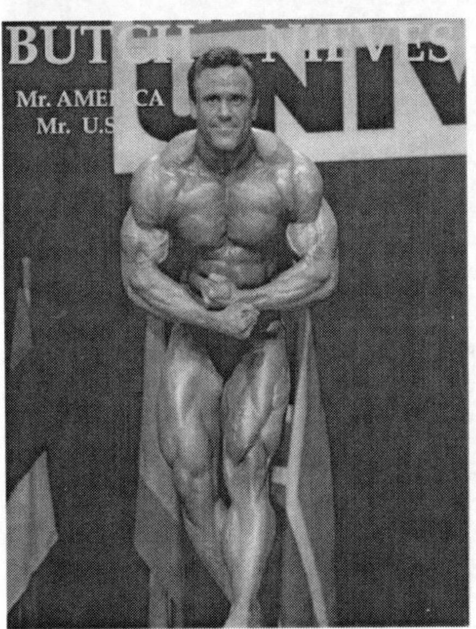

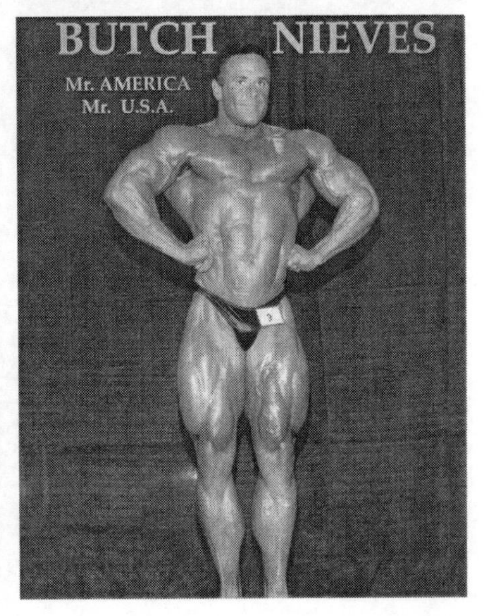
BUTCH NIEVES
Mr. AMERICA
Mr. U.S.A.

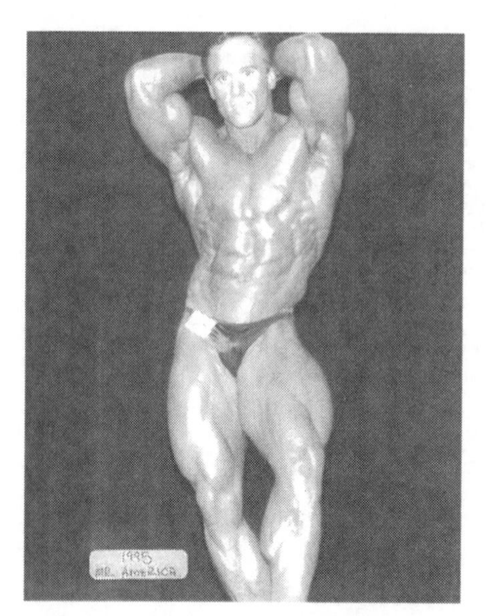
1995
MR. AMERICA

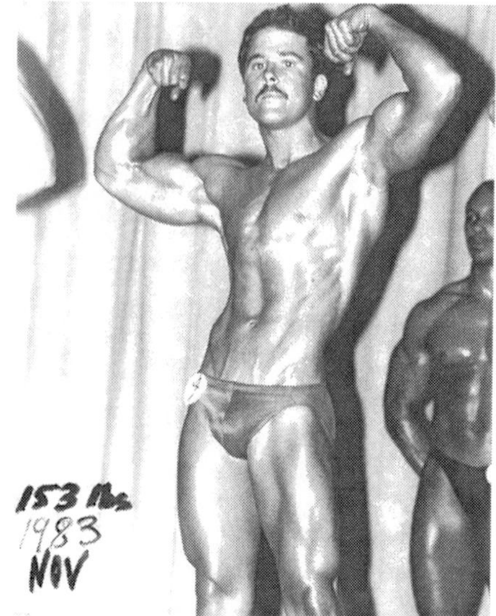
153 lbs
1983
NOV

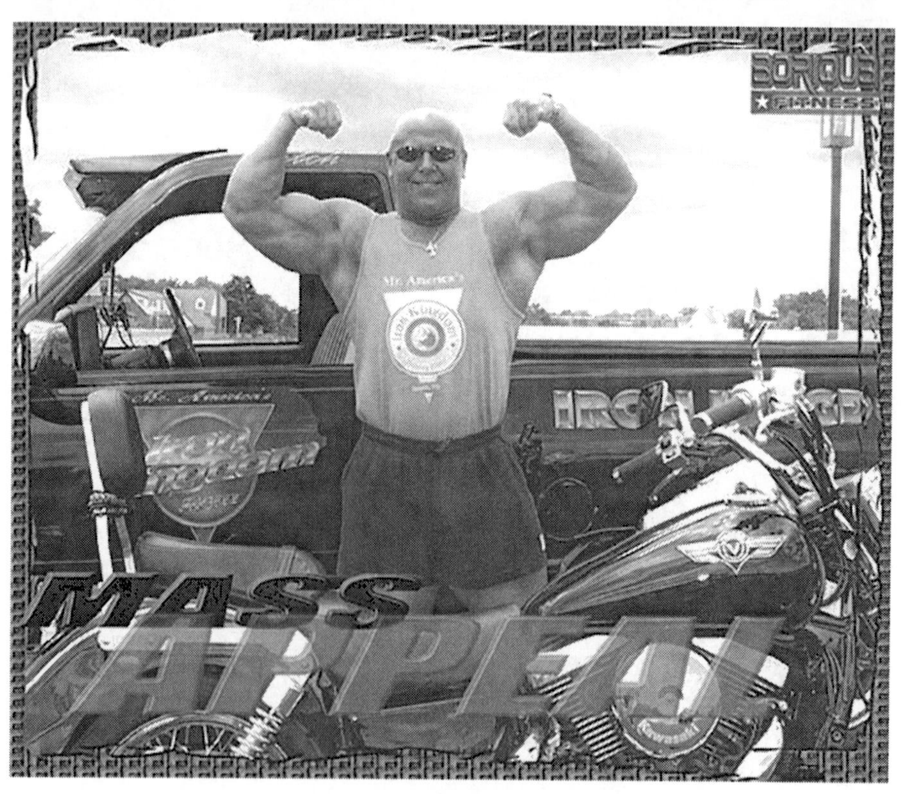
Mr. America's
MASS

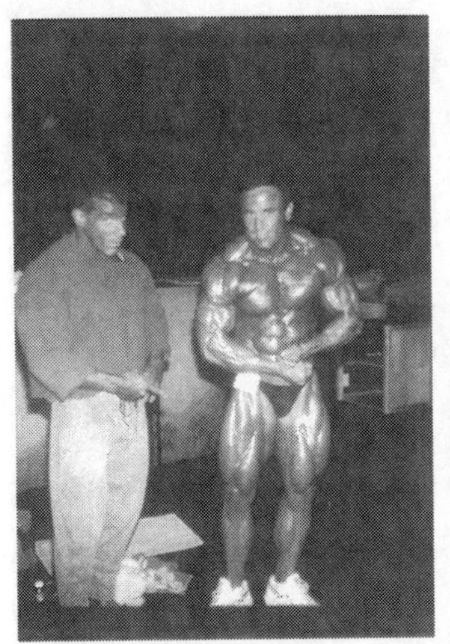

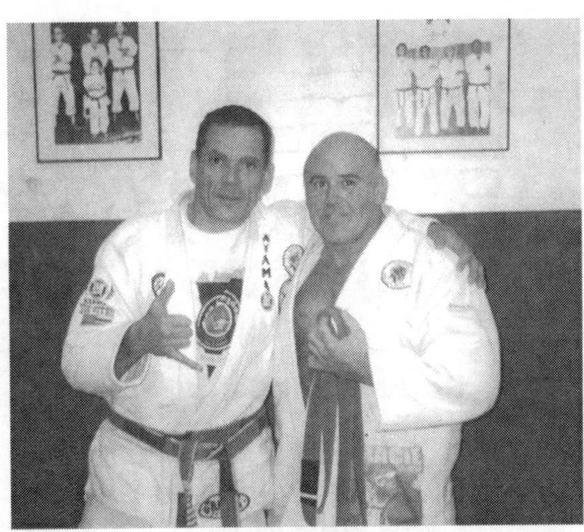

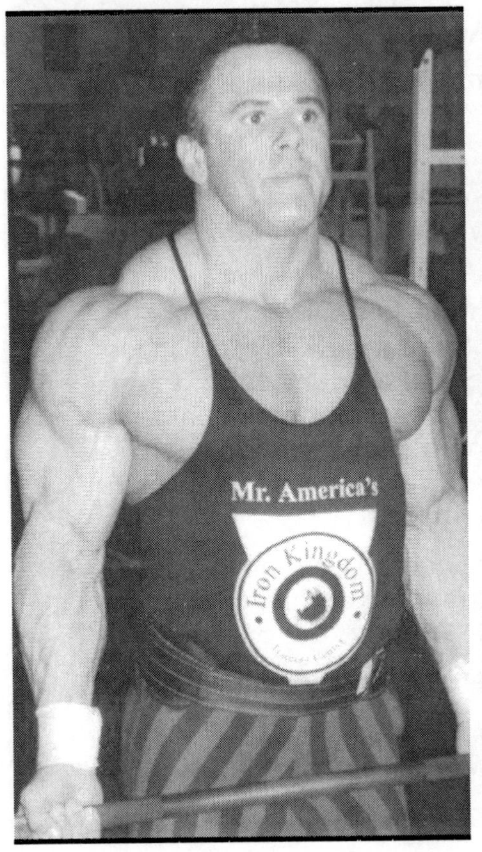
Mr. America's
Iron Kingdom

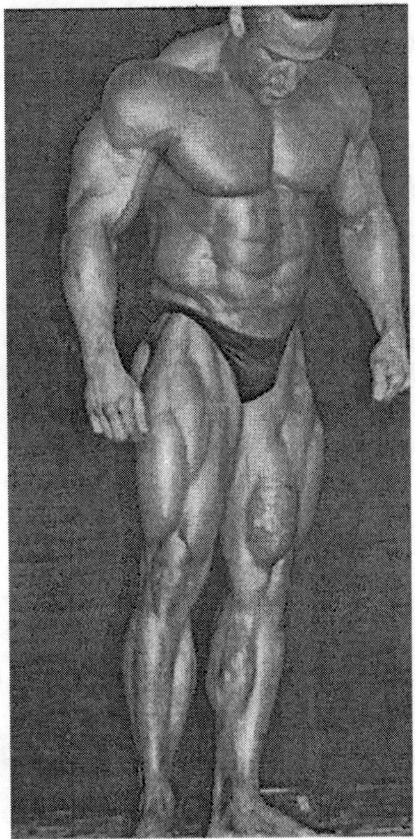

BE INSPIRED DAILY

Download these images in full color
for your smart phone or wall at

MrAmericasPersonalTraining.com/Resources

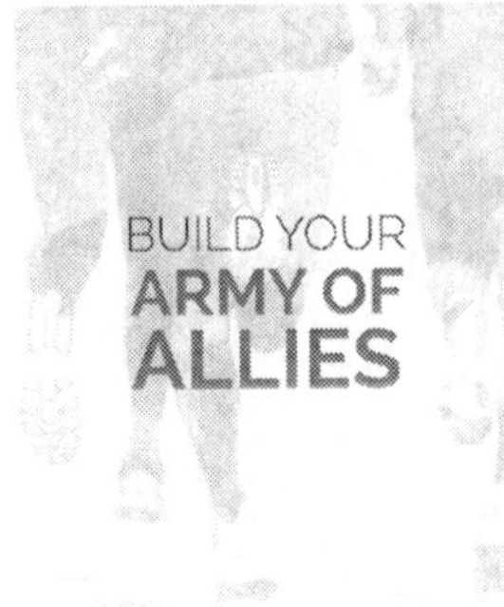

Our Biggest
Challenge Is
Developing
The Right Habits

BUTCH NIEVES
MR. AMERICA'S

TO CHOOSE
THE ACT IS
TO CHOOSE THE
CONSEQUENCES
OF THE ACT

BUTCH NIEVES
MR. AMERICA'S

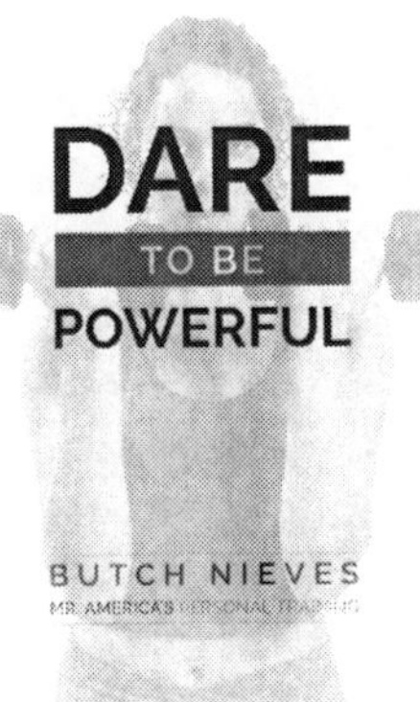

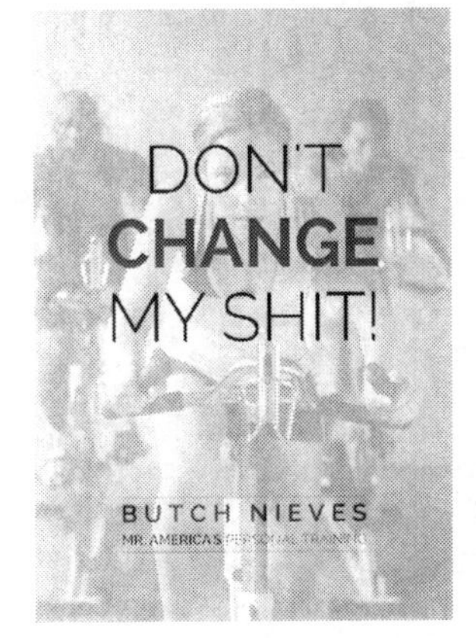

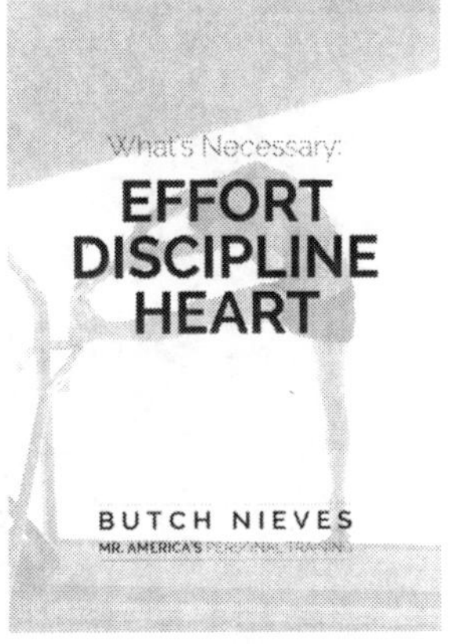

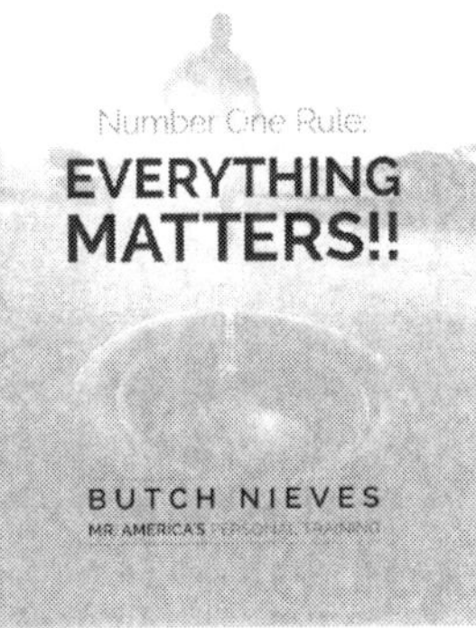

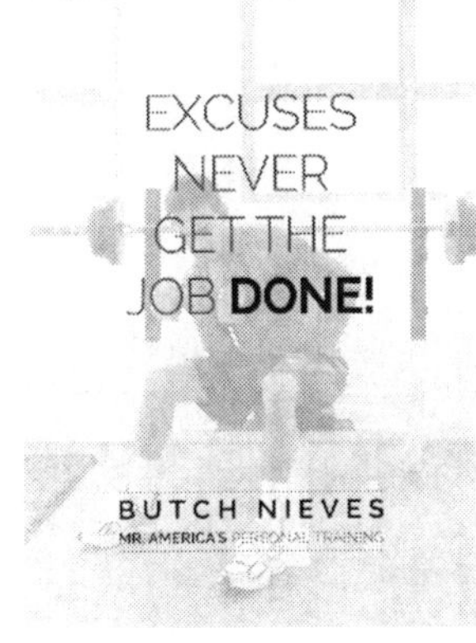

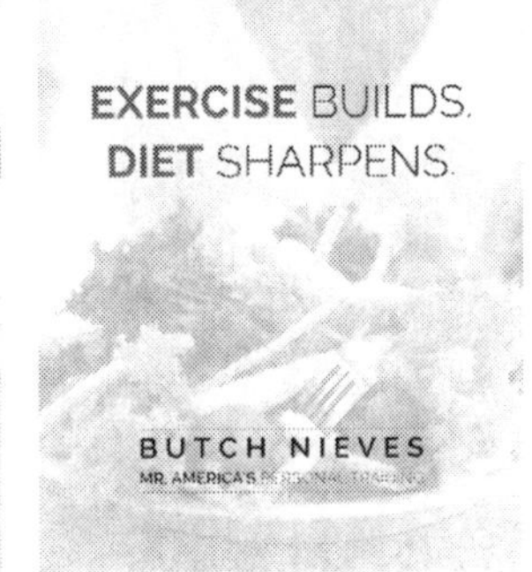

I Am Not A **BEAST**, I Am The One **You Call To Kill** The Beast

BUTCH NIEVES
MR. AMERICA'S PERSONAL TRAINING

IT'S NOT **WHAT YOU DO**, BUT HOW YOU **DO IT!**

BUTCH NIEVES
MR. AMERICA'S PERSONAL TRAINING

My **Job** Is To Get Thru Your **Mind** and Into Your **Heart**!

BUTCH NIEVES
MR. AMERICA'S PERSONAL TRAINING

LIFE IS NOT A MATH TEST!! IT'S ABOUT **HEART!**

BUTCH NIEVES
MR. AMERICA'S PERSONAL TRAINING

NO GUTS **NO** GLORY

BUTCH NIEVES
MR. AMERICA'S PERSONAL TRAINING

NO **PAIN**
NO **GAIN**
NO **BRAIN**

BUTCH NIEVES
MR. AMERICA'S PERSONAL TRAINING

PROGRESS
NOT PERFECTION

BUTCH NIEVES
MR. AMERICA'S PERSONAL TRAINING

TRAIN HARD. WIN EASY.

BUTCH NIEVES
MR. AMERICA'S PERSONAL TRAINING

WHEN YOU **GIVE UP** ON THE THINGS **YOU WANT**, THE THINGS YOU DON'T WANT **TAKE OVER**

BUTCH NIEVES
MR. AMERICA'S PERSONAL TRAINING

TRAIN **HARD**
TRAIN **SMART**
HAVE **FUN**

BUTCH NIEVES
MR. AMERICA'S PERSONAL TRAINING

CPSIA information can be obtained
at www.ICGtesting.com
Printed in the USA
LVOW10s1455081117
555505LV00027B/957/P

9 781946 533166